THE SACRED DISEASE

KRISTIN SEABORG, MD

GRΛVITY

Seattle WA 2015

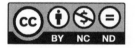
Cover Design by Greg Simanson
Edited by Justin Bog

Print ISBN 978-1-5137-0548-4
EPUB ISBN 978-1-5137-0599-6
Library of Congress Control Number: 2015955964

3 0646 00208 6738

For Andrew
Who always catches me.

Contents

Author's Note

To write this book, I relied on scrapbooks, journal entries, notes from my own medical record, interviews with friends and family members, research on topics related to epilepsy, and my memory. I've changed the names of many, but not all, characters in this book, and occasionally changed physical or historical details in order to preserve anonymity. The names of all of the patients encountered in this book have been changed and a few patients are composites of several different people I met over time. All details of my medical history, events and circumstances related to my own epilepsy, and interactions with my health care providers remain unchanged.

"People think epilepsy is divine simply because they don't have any idea what causes epilepsy. But I believe that we will someday understand what causes epilepsy, and at that moment, we will cease to believe that it's divine."
~ Hippocrates

Foreword

The latch on my bedroom window came loose years ago.

Night after night, I crept out my open window and perched on the worn yet rough shingles of the front porch roof. While I hovered above the peaceful suburban streets, I folded my legs and grew comfortable on my perch. Craning my neck, my gaze fixed on the twinkling lights of distant galaxies in the ephemeral night sky. On evenings when the moon brightened full of mystery, the rest of the sky dulled, became uniform grey-black, mired with shadows, and the stars hid from the overpowering moonlight.

When finally, and correctly, diagnosed with epilepsy at age eighteen, I decided to turn my life into a version of the full moon. If I could shine with enough brightness to draw attentive eyes to my outer shell, the darkness of the night within would remain unseen. I became a master of artificial brightness. Viewable only by those whom I trusted enough to learn the dark secret of my heart, the evening sky of my soul remained intact, brittle in its uniqueness, and something I could call my own.

But secrets smolder like an untended fire. My secret licked at my confidence and paralyzed with ironic movement, a flame's sputtering, while it left me mesmerized and unable to turn my eyes away. Well-hidden secrets, like mine, festered and grew until strong enough to threaten destruction of the stable foundation of the life I'd built.

One in twenty-six people worldwide and three million Americans suffer from epilepsy. By writing this book, I hope to give voice to my secret and help to change the tide of stigmatization.

"Three things cannot be hidden: the sun, the moon, and the truth."
~Buddha

Part I: The Student
1976—2002

1
1976

I DON'T REMEMBER the day that it all began.

My mother had told me the familiar story of my first seizure many times to provide a backdrop to my current life.

I was only sixteen months old and an active, happy toddler. On that ill-fated day in Springfield, Missouri, the skies were angry and congested with heavy grey clouds. My mother, grandmother, and I began the day with a trip to the local grocery store. I'm told that my keen toddler eyes found the most cherubic, soft-skinned shoppers and I pointed out every "baby" perched in the front baskets of passing shopping carts.

My mother remembers that my temperament changed abruptly moments after we returned home. My cheeks flushed red with a fever that quickly took on a life of its own. I was uninterested in my grandmother's diligent attempts to feed me lunch so instead she placed me in my crib to nap. Silently, my rapidly rising temperature hijacked my body and brain in what would be my first and most devastating seizure.

On that fateful day, my grandmother crept in to check on me shortly after she put me down to sleep. My mother heard the latch of my bedroom door click open followed by a suffocating blanket of silence. Then, like a cry of distress bellowed from the bottom of a crevasse, my grandmother screamed, "Jo-ney! Come quick!"

Mom ran to my bedroom and found Grandma struggling to cradle me in her arms. My body was simultaneously stiff as a tree trunk while captured by jarring, irregular movements. My grandmother and mother's synergistic maternal instincts took over as they hastily wrapped me in a warm blanket before they ran to the car to drive to the nearest hospital. There was no time to call an ambulance.

Seconds bled into minutes that crawled without end into almost an hour of unrelenting convulsing. As my seizure continued, my brain demanded extra blood flow and energy to feed the rampant and dysfunctional electrical activity. When the vulnerable areas deepest within my brain were overwhelmed, the most delicate structures in my developing neural circuits irreparably changed. The cascade of molecular events that followed left an indelible scar deep in my right temporal lobe.

Doctors were able to finally stop my seizure by placing me in a medically induced coma. Because my small body was overwhelmed by influenza—the infection that caused the initial fever—I remained lifeless on a ventilator in the St. Louis Children's Hospital for the next two weeks. A kaleidoscope of frightened family members, visitors, and medical staff stood by my side and delivered the protection and strong medicine that kept other seizures at bay. Tubes sprouted from my body like snakes from Medusa leading to ventilators, monitors, intravenous lines, and catheters that tethered me in a precarious cocoon of healing.

As my body slowly recovered from the illness, the medical instruments were peeled away like layers of onionskin until at last my spirited self re-emerged. When it was finally time to be discharged from the hospital, I ran playfully around the hospital room, dancing and chatting with the kind hospital staff members who'd taken care of me. Those who watched me dance and play thought that I'd endured the threat to my carefree childhood unscathed. But as we were leaving the hospital, the physician who cared for me through the whole ordeal warned, "This may not be the end of Kristin's seizures."

There's a picture in my mother's photo album from around this time. On the back of the picture, written in my grandmother's long, loopy handwriting: "Kristin Ann Gould, age 16 months. (Taken after her critical illness in April.)" I wore white coveralls with pink animal prints and a dainty pink shirt with ruffles. The sunlight ricocheted like pristine shards of glass on my shoulder-length sandy hair, and my eyes widened with curiosity. I sat on the shag carpet of my parents' living room grinning at something or someone out of camera range. I looked like the picture of health and wholesome American happiness.

*   *   *

When discharged from the hospital, I started taking the anti-epileptic medication phenobarbital to prevent further seizures. Though many begrudge taking daily medication, I loved it. My parents hid the small pills in a spoonful of chocolate pudding, applesauce, or ice cream. When Dad offered me a treat at the end of dinner, I anticipated a dollop of something sweet with a potent apple-seed-sized pill sandwiched within. I dutifully swallowed my powerful treats every day until I was five. After years without any evidence of seizures, it was time to consider stopping the medication.

Before he made any changes, my neurologist ordered an electroencephalogram (EEG) to ensure that my brain's electrical activity remained normal. The night prior to my EEG, my mother followed the doctor's instructions and kept me up hours past my usual bedtime. Mom and I watched TV and read stories until a late evening hour that I hadn't seen since the midnight feedings of infancy. I thought that the upcoming test—just like my daily treats—might be a lot of fun. My naive mind didn't understand the severity of the seizure years before or the gravity of what we were trying to avoid.

The morning of my EEG, I dressed in my favorite brown corduroy dress and patterned white tights before I bounced to school. I was eager to tell my kindergarten friends about what I watched on late night television. Their envy was obvious as I explained that I got to stay up *super late* and would go to the *hospital* for a test of my *brain waves.* None of my classmates had ever had a test of their brain waves before. I must be *really special.*

But at the end of my half-day of kindergarten, our teacher showed a Sesame Street movie about making friends. As soon as the lights dimmed and the shades were drawn, fatigue overwhelmed me. Moments after Elmo appeared on the screen, my head dropped back and I fell into a swift, deep sleep.

I awoke later with a stream of drool on my cheek, buzzing lights glaring overhead, and a room full of giggling children.

"You fell asleep!"

"Look at her drool!"

Another classmate pointed in my direction.

"I think she was snoring!"

A snickering room surrounded me.

My embarrassment and humiliation grew as I wiped the puddle of saliva off my face and rubbed the sleep out of my eyes. I looked around the room and found the bare projector screen blinking as my teacher watched me with a concerned expression. I remembered my late night with Mom, the upcoming EEG, and decided that brain wave tests couldn't be exciting, but they could be embarrassing. Medication transformed from unique and fun into something that made me different from my peers—strange, and to be ridiculed. For the first time in a lifetime, my seizures made me ashamed.

Later that week, I learned that my EEG results came back normal. Slowly, the doctor weaned my system off phenobarbital. Gradually, we forgot my first seizure and subsequent hospitalization, packed the memories away in dusty attic trunks full of unwanted things. Years passed before I learned what brewed within, biding its time.

2
1989

ONE DAY IN MY fourteenth year, the reset button of borrowed time ran down, and life as I knew it changed again. I joined my girlfriends at a local amusement park, and all of us enjoyed the warmth of the waning afternoon sun and the feeling of freedom that came with our teenage years. While the group of us walked from one ride to another, I stopped.

Anxious to visit all the biggest roller coasters before the end of the day, my longtime friend, Laura, said, "If we head this way, we can catch up with the other girls to ride the American Eagle. There's enough time to catch a few more rides before we have to meet my mom."

"Yeah, okay." My speech slurred; I tried to make sense of a pulsing presence that abruptly consumed me.

"Are you alright?" Laura asked. "Why are you doing that thing with your face?"

I ran my right hand through my hair, rhythmically, and swallowed repeatedly as a tremendous heat devoured me.

"Kristin, what's going on?"

As Laura's persistence changed to concern, I slowly returned to my normal self.

"Nothing. I'm okay. Let's get going." I followed the motion of her bright white Keds. A wave of headache and fatigue—a pattern I would learn to recognize—crashed over me as I bound ahead. An identical series of symptoms reoccurred while we waited in line to ride the pendulum-swinging ship.

Later that afternoon, I tried to explain the episode to my parents.

"So, you suddenly felt hot?" My mother looked at me with more than a little skepticism. "Did you drink enough water during the day? Perhaps you were dehydrated?"

"And I had this weird nervous feeling in my stomach."

My parents exchanged glances and tried to decipher my story. After a moment, my mother said, "I'll make an appointment with your doctor tomorrow."

The following day, I fidgeted while sitting next to my father in the pediatrician's waiting room. Stuffed animals and paper cutouts adorned the room that mimicked a children's playroom. I felt silly for being there at all. The light of the new day brought complete resolution of my symptoms, and I wondered if I could explain the episodes clearly enough. After a short wait, an assistant ushered us into Dr. Bradfield's office.

An elderly gentleman, Dr. Bradfield had been practicing pediatrics for more than thirty-five years. He had gentle hands with long, delicate fingers and an aged, welcoming face with rogue tufts of hair sprouting from his ears and nose. Dr. Bradfield had only seen me for a series of physicals and the occasional injury. Although he'd been my pediatrician since I was five, the medical records from my first seizure remained buried several states away, long forgotten in our minds. He looked at me with eyes cloudy with cataracts and asked, "What brings you here today, Kristin?"

With my father's quiet, comforting presence at my side, I tried to describe the episodes at the amusement park.

Uncertainty marched across his face.

"Hot...nervous...swallowing...headache...weird stomach thing..." I pieced the symptoms together in the best narrative I could.

"So your stomach was really bothering you." He interrupted my rambling description of what I'd endured. "Looks like we have to do an exam."

Dr. Bradfield beckoned me to lie supine on the exam table, and the color rose in my pubescent cheeks. My father averted his eyes when Dr. Bradfield raised my shirt, squashed my abdomen, and performed a rectal exam to collect a stool sample. I was thoroughly embarrassed.

"Well, your exam is normal today, Kristin. Perhaps the greasy food at the amusement park got the best of you?" he chuckled jovially. "I think the symptoms you describe are from a sour stomach."

Dr. Bradfield returned to his desk and wrote a note with a shaky hand. He passed the paper to my dad. "Next time Kristin experiences these symptoms, give her one teaspoon of Maalox and she should feel better."

My dad murmured assent while Dr. Bradfield left the room ahead of us.

I walked to the car behind my father, muttering in frustration. *Sour stomach? Maalox? Was that really all that was going on?*

After the initial event in the amusement park, hundreds of episodes identical to the first appeared. They occurred at anytime and anywhere, while sitting in American History class, when doing homework, in the middle of the night, or when squeezed next to my make-up laden teenage friends in the backseat of their cars. Although largely unpredictable, I searched for subtle patterns to my symptoms so I could do my best to mask the events.

I found that the events almost always occurred just before my menstrual cycle and that they always started with a sense of eerie familiarity as if I was reliving something that I dreamt the night before. One afternoon in Spanish class I studied an innocuous pink flyer hanging on the bulletin board. While I stared at the flyer, the simple piece of paper began to look strikingly familiar. Before long, my thoughts dulled as I succumbed to the heat, swallowing, and familiar rhythmic hand movements of another episode.

At a lack for words to describe what was going on, I came to call the events *Weirds* because, simply, I felt weird when I was having one. When my classmates noticed my smacking lips and repetitive hand movements, some giggled, while a few of them sneered.

"Are you having another *Weird*, Kristin? Or are you just trying to get out of pom-pom practice today?"

"Kristin, can you even hear me? Earth to Kristin!"

I heard everything during the events but had limited ability to respond appropriately. While the episodes grew in intensity and frequency, I fostered a growing sense of shame about the embarrassing and unusual behaviors that were beyond my control.

To avoid laughter and ridicule, I hid myself when I felt a *Weird* coming so no one had to know. At times I turned my head toward a textbook so others would assume I was reading. When I wasn't sitting in class, I wandered out of view to a corner or behind a tree whenever I felt the preceding aura of déjà vu. In the week preceding my menstrual cycle each month, there were days when I had ten episodes or more. I became skilled at fiercely hiding the monster that was gaining strength within.

I didn't talk about the episodes to anyone. I was afraid another doctor's visit would lead to another joke about greasy food and Maalox, and I was reluctant to admit that my carefully constructed life was slipping beyond control. For the next four years, I did my best to predict bad days, hide when I felt an aura, and act as if nothing was different. Like every flawed plan, it was only a matter of time before my secret was exposed.

3
1993

THE SPRING OF MY eighteenth year filled with excitement, new beginnings, and a multitude of activity. Our high school produced *The Wizard of Oz*, and I played the part of Auntie Em. I loved the feeling of being on stage and acting as if I were in a different place at a different time. Whether my companions were flying monkeys or disturbing *Weirds*, I was adept at feigning normalcy. Between play rehearsals, college preparation, and social events, I found little time to sleep.

The senior class held a Red Cross blood drive, and I was eager to participate. A woman with long hair and a Wanda name-tag pinned to her blouse sat in the makeshift office and asked dozens of screening questions.

"Were you a recipient of blood products prior to 1980?" Her tone became demanding, meant to intimidate and pull honesty from her subjects.

"No."

"Do you have a history of anemia?"

"No."

"Have you ever had a seizure?"

I paused. "Well, there was that one when I was a baby and sick with a fever."

Wanda scratched some notes on her paper and then lifted her eyes to meet mine. "Sounds like you're OK to go then." With a whisk of the paper and clap of the clipboard, she swung out of her chair and led me to a seat next to a nurse with a needle.

The task of donating blood was uneventful. After the nurse removed the needle from my arm, I felt weak like the rest of my classmates. That afternoon, however, I pushed myself through several small episodes with the swallowing and warmth that'd now become as familiar to me as dark alleys to thieves. When my American History teacher noted my glassy-eyed gaze during one of these events, she sent me to the school nurse for evaluation.

"What's going on, Kristin?"

The last time I saw the school nurse was after I jammed my finger playing basketball my freshman year.

"I gave blood today. I'm just feeling a little tired, I guess."

The school nurse nodded understanding. "We've seen several kids like you today." She fished in the nearby refrigerator for some juice. "Why don't you drink some of this and rest for a while."

I lay down on the turquoise vinyl bed lined with sterile paper. The shapeless pillow smelled like antiseptic, and the paper lining crinkled every time I moved. Still, it was only seconds before I drifted to sleep.

After a while, the nurse gently jostled my leg. "Are you ready to go back to class now?"

I had no idea how long I'd been resting, but I felt better. "Sure." I sat up quickly. "I've got calculus during eighth hour."

"Take it easy, Kristin," the nurse warned. "You still look a little pale."

I sauntered down the empty hallway back to class.

At the end of the day, I walked out with a pack of friends. I listened half-heartedly as my girlfriends chatted amicably about their prom dresses, latest boyfriends, and other assorted school gossip. We ambled toward the parking lot and soon I was conscious of the presence of another aura. This time, the familiar déjà vu moved on to abdominal discomfort and rising heat, but didn't abate. When I couldn't make sense of things any more, I tried to beckon, "Help me!"

Then everything went black.

I woke up in the bay of an ambulance, lights pulsing, brightening walls lined with labeled boxes, and a stranger's face hovering directly above mine.

"Do you know where you are?" the stranger asked.

I shook my head.

"You're in an ambulance. You've had a grand mal seizure."

I wasn't completely sure what a grand mal seizure was, but I vaguely remembered that the main character of a popular TV show had one. During a memorable recent episode, they depicted the teenage main character violently convulsing on the ground with limbs wild, saliva spewing, and a harsh, feral guttural sound emanating from within. Through my foggy consciousness, I imagined what the scene at my high school must've been like. I pictured a crowd of students, faces aghast, as they watched me twitch and clench uncontrollably. I shuddered in humiliation as I envisioned my own saliva foaming on my lips while my arms and legs moved as if possessed.

What would they think of me now?

I wished I could return to the stage with my fellow Wizard of Oz cast-mates and pretend I was someone else. The fantasy of Auntie Em was much preferable to my present reality, especially when life wasn't following my internally prepared script.

I spent four days in the hospital after that grand mal seizure. I acquiesced to scans and studies, EKGs and EEGs. Finally, discharge day came along with a diagnosis of "likely seizure disorder."

Pictures of me after I returned home from Elmbrook Hospital show me propped on my family's black vinyl couch with blankets piled high, and my friends clustered around. I held a stuffed bunny, a season-appropriate get-well gift from a friend at church. Fresh flowers on the coffee table shared an ebullient "Get Well!" printed on the attached card. My girlfriends leaned around me and into each other.

Behind their fixed smiles, they hid their confusion and discomfort. The camera lens couldn't hide the fact that I wasn't myself. In the photo, my hair remained disheveled and my eyes were accompanied by the dusky ringed hue of exhaustion. My arms clenched tightly and protectively around my torso and the stuffed toy. I temporarily lost the spark that built the very foundation of youth and independence.

My release from the hospital didn't mean the end of diagnostic tests and procedures. Because the tests done in the hospital hadn't led to a definitive diagnosis, my neurologist, Dr. Cook, recommended a continuous outpatient EEG. For this procedure, I was instructed to wear the EEG electrodes and attached wires for three days. I also was required to carry a large computer-monitoring unit with an attached extension cord at all times. The neurology team hoped to capture a tracing of atypical electrical activity to confirm a diagnosis of epilepsy.

Several days later, my mom followed Dr. Cook's orders and took me to the outpatient neurology clinic. Sandy, the EEG technician on duty that day, made me feel welcome as best as she could. As her cold fingers moved quickly around my head, she placed each electrode and then cemented them to my scalp with glue, rubbing harshly with the pointed tip of the glue bottle each time it met my skin. I cringed and cowered from the sharp pinch of the glue tip but this only led Sandy to pull my head back in place by my hair. I felt relief only when all nineteen electrodes were in place and the glue was returned to its safe spot in the drawer.

After Sandy attached the cords from the electrodes to a central monitoring device, I reached down to collect my things and prepared to go. Sandy lifted an open hand to my face and instructed, "Wait." I sat back down.

With a flourish, Sandy produced an enormous roll of gauze as big and fluffy as a roll of toilet paper. She methodically wrapped the gauze around and around my wired head until I sported a two-foot tall turban that piled high into the air. She wrapped a long loop of gauze around my chin for a final touch before she declared the job finished.

And I was supposed to go to school this way?

Fortunately, my parents accepted my extension cord and electrodes as an excuse not to attend school. Still, I went to piano lessons and my friend's house while dressed like a wired Sikh. With familial kindness, my parents and I laughed at my new hairdo and we found plenty of ways to joke about the fact that I needed to remain attached to the wall at all times by a ten-foot leash of electrical cord.

"Just need to plug myself in," I said with a goofy smile.

"Kristin, why don't you rest and recharge your batteries?" My dad suggested as he held the plug to the monitoring unit in his hand. My dad used his gentle manner and quick wit to help me relax and not feel self-conscious.

Laughing at my own jokes about my extension cord and portable computer unit hid brewing unease. Despite my best efforts to appear "normal," the turban and electrodes revealed my mounting fear of vulnerability

Three long days later, Sally's frigid fingers removed my electrodes and wires. I left the extension cord and large computer-recording unit with the neurologist and fled to pom-pom practice. With the flip of a switch, I was once again a healthy high school senior. College was only months away, and I was ready to leave seizures behind.

Later that week, I visited Dr. Cook's office to discuss the results of my outpatient EEG. His impeccable mustache and three-piece suit contrasted with his office overflowing with models of the human brain. He delivered his diagnosis while standing next to the door holding a thin paper chart in his hand. His mustache bounced as he talked, and his steel-rimmed glasses reflected the florescent lights so that his eyes were replaced with circular mirrors.

"Although you didn't have any reportable events during the EEG tracing," he said, "we can see some baseline electrical charges that are consistent with epilepsy."

At the age of eighteen, I was no more familiar with epilepsy than I was with the foreign policy of China. I vaguely remembered the stories about my seizure during childhood but our family had filed that event safely away into our small collection of unpleasant memories. Although I'd been experiencing *Weirds* for several years, I had no idea that those episodes were seizures.

"What does that mean?" My mother sat beside me, equally at sea.

Dr. Cook sat down and grabbed a nearby pamphlet. "Take this home for review." He handed the thin pamphlet to my mother. "Epilepsy is the diagnosis given to patient who've had two or more unprovoked seizures. Based on your history and EEG findings, we should start you on an anti-epileptic medication to decrease the chance of more episodes."

He smoothed his mustache, took a breath, and plowed on before my mother could voice the question forming on her lips. "I'd like you to start taking carbamazepine today, Kristin. Carbamazepine is an anti-epileptic medication that's used in treatment of complex partial seizures with secondary generalization."

My mind swam. *Complex partial seizures? Secondary generalization?*

Dr. Cook looked at us, his eyes buggy behind their glass covers. "This medicine has a chance of decreasing the number of your white blood cells, so we'll have to see you for monthly lab draws until things are stabilized. It might make you feel a little tired when you first start taking it, but things will normalize soon enough."

He smoothed his mustache again. "Please make an appointment with me in one month."

He rose from his seat abruptly and whisked out the door. We had a pamphlet and a diagnosis, but few answers. While my mom arranged my next appointment at the reception desk, I scanned the other pamphlets in the waiting room. I picked a small library of material related to epilepsy. *Women with Epilepsy, Living with Epilepsy, Your Epilepsy Medications,* etc. I searched for guidance in small, two-page pamphlets written at the eighth-grade level. Time would quickly teach me that no amount of information could navigate the tumultuous path of a life with seizures.

Once I collected all the pamphlets I could find, I had a moment to spare before my mom finished scheduling future appointments. I sat down again in Dr. Cook's waiting room and observed the other patients. A little girl in a wheelchair held tightly to her mother's sleeve with twisted fingers. Next to her, an older boy twitched and gazed unconvincingly at the book in front of him. Across the room, another teenage girl spoke jovially with her companion but had periodic moments of hoarseness and a visible square lump underneath the skin of her neck.

Almost immediately, I separated myself from the other kids. Although we shared a reason to be in the neurologist's office, I convinced myself that they looked and acted vastly different than me. Little did I know how similar we were.

When we walked out of the doctor's office that afternoon, the sweet smell of the warming spring air struck me. Pregnant buds dotted the tree branches and green shoots burst through the cool soil. The days lengthened, and the world renewed around me with majesty and grace. While we ambled down the cracked grey path to the car, I made a decision from a deep sense of calm: I would learn to live with this new, bold, disruptive companion, but I would *never* let epilepsy define me. I wouldn't let seizures alter my goals and expectations.

The arrogance of my eighteen-year-old self was breathtaking.

In that moment, my resolve to fight seizures deepened with every step. I crumpled the informative pamphlets with gusto and threw them into a nearby garbage can. Immediately, I felt lighter and empowered in spite of my new prescriptions and diagnosis.

I convinced myself I was no different than the person who had donated blood a few weeks ago.

I convinced myself I was free.

*　*　*

The next several months were a whirlwind of neurology visits, blood tests to check medication levels, and the bittersweet activities of a graduating senior. In subsequent visits, my neurologist determined that the *Weirds* I'd experienced since age fourteen were complex partial seizures. I learned that complex partial seizures are periods of irregular brain activity that involve part of the brain and cause impairment, but not loss, of consciousness. Dr. Cook sat at his desk in his three-piece suit and fiddled with his gold cuff links when he delivered the news that ten to twelve daily seizures once or twice a month could actually eventually *form* damaging electrical pathways in my brain, a process called kindling.

Kindling is the neuroscientist's word to describe the molecular changes in brain structure and function that occur when experimental animals suffer repeated seizures. In other words, recurrent seizures that follow the same electrical pathway create new, easily excitable networks that change the landscape of the brain just as a river slowly carves a path through rocks to create a canyon.

As early as 1968, neuroscientist Graham Goddard noted that repeated stimulation of certain portions of the brain in normal rats eventually led to permanent increased propensity toward seizures.[1] Later studies determined that as increasing numbers of seizures were evoked, animal brains showed a pattern of neuronal cell loss and formation of irregular cellular connections.[2] Left untreated or resistant to medications, these recurrent seizures could have detrimental effects on a patient's cognitive function, mood, or both.[3]

While intellectually fascinated with what Dr. Cook described, I became afraid of what this might mean for me.

Would I live with seizures forever?

*   *   *

E

Documentation of patients affected by epilepsy can be found dating back to the beginning of recorded human history. During the Vedic period in India, as early as 4500-1500 BC, epilepsy was described as "apasmara" or "loss of consciousness." The ancient Babylonians recorded accounts of as many different seizure types as we recognize today on tablets that date back to 2000 BC. Considered a divine punishment for sinners, the Babylonians were one of the first cultures to claim a supernatural nature to epilepsy by associating each seizure type with an evil spirit or god.

In the 5th century BC, the Father of Medicine, Hippocrates, coined the term "seleniazetai" to describe people with epilepsy because they were believed to be affected by the moon god, Selene, and the phases of the moon. Hippocrates' term inspired the Latinized label "moonstruck" or "lunatic" that later arose to describe epileptics. However, Hippocrates was the first to attribute the etiology of epilepsy to brain dysfunction. He called epilepsy the "great disease," thus creating the origin for the term "grand mal." While Hippocrates believed that epilepsy had a physiologic cause, the perception that epilepsy was something beyond a spiritual problem or a curse wasn't accepted until the 18th and 19th centuries.

Despite the historical view that patients with epilepsy were dysfunctional and unable to lead productive lives, there were multiple famous historical figures who lived with epilepsy. Julius Cesar, Peter the Great of Russia, Händel, Berlioz, Pope Pius IX, and the writer Fodor Dostoevsky were all reported to have had epilepsy. George Washington's stepdaughter, Patsy, had a history of seizures. The success and prominence of these few, however, did little to change the public perception that epileptics were to be feared and avoided.

4

WHILE I FINISHED my last year of high school, my eldest brother completed his first year of medical school at the University of Wisconsin. Jon spent hours each day in the Gross Anatomy lab where he learned the intricate details of the human body by dissecting a cadaver donated to the medical school. Shortly after I was diagnosed with epilepsy, Jon invited my parents and me to visit the Anatomy lab so we could learn about the human body firsthand.

Jon greeted us at the entrance of the circa-1960s building that housed the University of Wisconsin Medical School. The thick, concrete slabs and stately columns adorning the building made me feel as if we were entering a large tomb. We passed students playing ping-pong in the hallway and others chatting around a table in the library as we made our way down to the basement anatomy lab. Jon waved to several of his classmates and led us to the far basement corner of the building that held the cadavers.

Before he opened the thick, impermeable doors to the gross anatomy lab, Jon looked at me affectionately with his characteristic lopsided smile and said, "Are you ready for this?"

The pungent smell of formaldehyde washed over us. Ahead there were eight stainless steel tanks, each propped on three-foot poles with wheels. There were dirty lab coats strewn over the nearby lockers and chairs and open anatomy books scattered on almost every flat surface around each tank. Jon picked up a coat with small flecks of material—could that be flesh?—scattered up the arms and over the breast pocket. He was completely comfortable in his official aromatic attire. Methodically, he opened the two awkward steel doors that concealed his cadaver in the tank. I closed my eyes and braced my arm against a nearby tank in case I fainted when it was time to see the long-dead human body.

"Our cadaver died when he was 82," Jon explained. "I know that he had a wife, but they don't disclose much else of his family or medical history for privacy reasons."

Instead of fainting, I was overcome with awe when Jon talked about his cadaver. I opened my eyes and the sheer mystery of the partially dissected body in front of me triggered something deep within. What was previously walking and talking flesh had become an intricate puzzle to be scrutinized and studied. In the midst of my teenage musings about what outfit to wear and how I would re-adjust to life with epilepsy, I hadn't thought much about my ultimate goals in life beyond high school.

Jon handed me some opaque gloves and nodded his assent when I stretched them over my fingers. I stepped closer to the cadaver that rested in the silver bed of eternal slumber. My breath caught as I reached out to touch the heart of the man who'd so generously donated his body to science. I caressed his stiff, lifeless hands and wondered what his years on earth had been like. Had he been a father? A grandfather? How did he spend his days?

A portion of the cadaver's skull had been removed to reveal the brain. I admired the magical gelatinous tissue lined with ridges and valleys that rested perfectly inside the skull like a cluster of overfed worms. It was hard to believe that such a simple-appearing, unassuming organ was the mainframe and data warehouse for the entire human body. I imagined where the electrical currents would ebb and flow across the microscopic synapses within the inconspicuous mass of tissue. I marveled at how even one small electrical glitch could evoke a powerful storm and disrupt the entire system.

I moved gingerly from one part of the body to the next. Unexpectedly, I found my home. My previous thoughts about studying to become a teacher or a writer evaporated into thin air. I wanted to study and understand the temple of creation in front of me.

Shortly after my trip to the Gross Anatomy lab, I applied for a program at the University of Wisconsin targeted at motivated Wisconsin high school students. If accepted into the Medical Scholars program, I would have to maintain a high GPA and take a core group of pre-med classes. If admitted to the program and if I could achieve the defined undergraduate goals, I was guaranteed a spot at the University of Wisconsin Medical School. Like a watched pot set to boil and about to roll over, I waited for an acceptance letter. Within weeks, the golden ticket arrived. UW-Madison accepted me into the undergraduate class of 1997 and the UW Medical School's class of 2001.

Like my brother, I was going to be a doctor.

*   *   *

E

Until as recently as the 20th century, people with epilepsy were viewed with fear, stigmatization, suspicion, and as social outcasts. British neurologist Rajendra Kale wrote in 1997:

> "The history of epilepsy can be summarized as 4000 years of ignorance, superstition, and stigma followed by 100 years of knowledge, superstition and stigma. Knowing that seizures result from sudden, excessive, abnormal electrical charges of a set of neurons in the brain has done little to dispel misunderstanding about epilepsy in most of the world."[4]

From Hippocrates' time to the early 20th century, epilepsy was thought to be contagious. Greeks and Romans who lived during the 4th and 5th centuries BC believed that epilepsy was caused by the presence of demons in a person. If an epileptic touched another, they feared the demon would spread unless the unaffected spat immediately.

In contrast to the early Greeks and Romans, nobility and clergy living in the Middle Ages believed that epilepsy wasn't a disease but instead a sign of prophetic powers and great intelligence. However, a 1494 handbook on witch hunting written by two Dominican friars, *The Malleus Mallificarum*, stated that the way to identify a witch was by the presence of seizures. This notion led to the death and torture of many epileptics who were thought to be witches.

A hospital for the "paralyzed and epileptic" was established in London in 1859, and epilepsy colonies were formed for the care and employment of epileptics in Denmark, England, Germany, Holland, Norway, and Switzerland. People with epilepsy were locked in mental hospitals in wards separate from the mentally ill, in effort to protect the mentally ill patients from contracting seizures.

5

EVEN THOUGH SPRING finally rolled around, I felt as if I should settle down for a long, subdued rest as my doctor continued to increase the dose of my anti-epileptic medication. Dr. Cook explained that he would start the medication at a low dose and gradually increase it to a higher level as my body learned to tolerate it. I accepted the warning that the medication might make me feel a little groggy, but I couldn't prepare for the full force of fatigue that hit me head-on. I had enough energy to go to school and do a small amount of homework, but then I'd collapse into a deep sleep for ten to twelve hours each night. I wondered how I'd ever make it through college living in a cognitive fog.

I sought comfort and peace wherever I could. I rested in the field behind our neighborhood where the wind played music as it blew through the reeds. I took refuge at the park down the street where the voices of children echoed like ghosts. I searched for renewal at the Lutheran church a few blocks away where I took a summer job as a church organist.

From my clumsy grammar school days through the awkwardness of adolescence, my long-time piano teacher, Mrs. Busse, taught me with the same firm affirmation and gentle guidance. She sat in the corner chair of her living room every week for ten years and listened as I poked at the wrong keys and eventually emerged as a respectable piano player. With steadfast diligence, Mrs. Busse set the metronome to click faster and faster while my fingers gained agility and speed. Her kind brown eyes smiled as she said sternly, week after week, "You can do better, Kristin."

Mrs. Busse was also the organist at our neighborhood church. As my piano skills improved, she declared that it was time I learn to play the organ as well. Eventually, I was asked to fill in as the church organist for a summer when she took medical leave.

I rehearsed for the Sunday services when the church was empty in the afternoons. I let myself in with my own key and enjoyed the cool quiet of the sanctuary. I loved to turn the organ up as loud as possible, and I basked in the sheer joy of the music that eclipsed whatever was troubling me.

On an afternoon filled with frustration and lassitude, I went to the church for some time to rehearse and think. After I turned on the lights and set up the hymnal, I put all my weight into my right foot to turn the volume pedal up as high as it could go. I played through the hymn "Blest Are They" several times, and, tentative at first, sang along for the last few rounds. When I finished and pulled my fingers off the keys, the cavernous sanctuary vibrated with sound for a few magical moments. I sensed a presence in the room so strongly that I turned to look at the doors to make sure that no one was there.

Once I affirmed I was still alone, I whispered with a shaking voice: "God, is that you?" The silence remained, but I found my answer in the quiet calm of the ethereal presence. I felt at peace for the first time in months. Maybe it was true that I was never alone. Perhaps omnipotence was something more than an esoteric principle I was taught in Sunday school.

My God wasn't always noticeable in the masses of a church service or in the din of a hospital hallway or clinic entryway. God was easiest for me to find in quiet and in spare spaces. If I was attentive, I could hear God in the quiet of a setting sun, or in the moments before light breaks on a day unknown. As the years marched on and mounting obstacles arose, I never came to question God's love for me, although I certainly might have. Instead I chose to count my blessings, every one of them. He was the composer of the musical laughter of my family and the orchestrator of the beauty around us. God made himself known, omnipresent in the deafening silence that screamed as I woke from each grand mal seizure and battled to understand the world again.

6

AS THE SUMMER of 1993 inched on, the oppressive mental fog lifted as I gradually acclimated to my anti-epileptic medication. Six months passed since my last seizure and epilepsy felt like a burden that didn't belong to me anymore. Full of energy, I filled an entire room in my parent's house with supplies while I prepared for college.

The morning I left for college quickly became scorching hot. By eight A.M. the humidity hung in the thickening air surrounding my parents' SUV. We loaded bag after bag into the car, and Dad and I soon worked up a sweat that held fast to our skin instead of evaporating. Regardless of the temperature, excitement grew as I began my journey to the University of Wisconsin.

My mother came out of the house before our scheduled departure and turned away in effort to hide her tear-streaked face. Her puffy eyes exuded kindness and worry as she methodically ticked down the mental list of things all incoming students were expected to bring to campus that day. "Do you have your sheets and comforter?"

"Yes."

"Your address book and contact information?"

"Yes."

"Your clothes and winter coat and robe?"

"Mo-ooom!" I couldn't hide my exasperation.

"Do you have your medicine, Kristin? You know that's really important."

I'd already packed two months' worth of carbamazepine to tide me over until I found a pharmacy in Madison. A day of missed medication could trigger almost immediate seizures. "Yes, mom, I have that, too. Now, can we get going?"

Since we had enough gear to fill two cars, my older brother Paul volunteered to drive with me to Madison. My parents followed closely behind in the packed second car to form a collegiate caravan. Paul used the 90-minute drive to instruct in what he felt was a constructive way, to prepare me for college in a brotherly manner. When we pulled off the interstate and onto campus, Paul did his best to both embarrass me and ease the tension of the landmark day.

"Kristin Gould is here!" he yelled out through open windows. "Hey, everyone! Look over here. Kristin Gould has arrived on campus!" Passers-by looked at our car and laughed. Laughter from strangers only fueled Paul's ebullience and made him louder. I shrunk out of my seat and giggled on the floor of the car. "Paul Gould's little sister is here! Look out everybody, here she comes!"

Thankfully, we found my dormitory in a short amount of time. Sellery Hall, a thick, concrete building, appeared impervious to whatever behavioral insults rambunctious college freshmen could offer. Paul and Dad parked the cars in tight non-spaces close to the crowded entrance, and a cheery Resident Assistant leapt out the front door offering welcome wishes. The RA wore a sweaty Bucky Badger shirt and carried a crumpled list of freshman names on a bright yellow clipboard.

"Name?" He said this with an air of authority.

"Kristin Gould."

"Oh! We've got you right here. Follow me!" It felt like his enthusiasm grew stronger as he bounced into the elevator. He escorted me to the ninth floor and down the hall to a marred wooden door.

"This," he exclaimed, opening the door with a flourish, "is your room!"

Mom, Dad, Paul and I gazed at the nine by sixteen foot space drained of both color and character. We couldn't help but laugh. My new shared home was smaller than my old bedroom, but despite the cramped quarters, I couldn't wait to move in.

My roommate arrived soon after with another energetic family and two times as much luggage. Jasmine had long, flowing blonde hair and a wide, friendly smile outlined by fresh pink lipstick. She came from a small Wisconsin farming town but had plenty of Big City experience from visiting her older friends in Madison. We clicked right away.

My freshman year at the University of Wisconsin soon filled with books, introductions to friends, and newfound freedom. Because my neurologist warned that drinking alcohol could provoke seizures, I made friends with quiet, introspective students who spent hours daydreaming in coffee shops or exploring the world outside our small cocoon of campus.

I met Jeff, Tim, and Lisa in my freshman expository writing class. Jeff grew up in Hackensack, New Jersey, but his soft voice and gentle manner fit none of the slick stereotypes I had of freshman from the East coast. He had soulful brown eyes and an infectious laugh accompanied by a biting sense of humor. On the other hand, Tim, who grew up in Manhattan, enjoyed making provocative statements and wore an expression of feigned indifference to mask his sensitivity. The constant glint in his eye revealed both his intelligence and mischievousness. Lisa was the second of three children who came from a town near Ames, Iowa. Her Midwestern upbringing molded her into a trusting, kind woman who saw the best in everyone. Together we formed a tight, loyal crew.

Tim, Jeff, Lisa and I spent countless hours together during our first year at UW. We visited local Madison attractions and took tours of the Veteran's Museum, the Children's Museum, and the state Capitol. We huddled around the lava lamps in our dorm rooms and dreamt about what our futures would bring. Tim hoped to become a politician. Jeff was studying to be a journalist. Lisa wanted to be a teacher. I longed to become a doctor.

The combination of new friends, new opportunities, and a promising future made my freshman year a magical time. I felt well, my admission to medical school was secured, and I had the freedom to head in which-ever direction I chose. With hopes and dreams piled miles higher than my small cache of worries, there was no way I could lose.

*   *   *

E

In Nazi Germany in the 1920s, sterilization sur-geries were performed on patients with epilepsy to ensure they didn't reproduce. In the US, people with epilepsy were forbidden to marry in seventeen states until 1956, but repeal of this law led to the encouragement of sterilization of epileptics in eighteen states.[5]

Throughout history, epileptics have fought against fear, stigma, and misunderstanding. Perhaps the most damning statement referring to the stigma associated with epileptics was written by Dr. Eugene Billod in 1882. In some circumstances, it still applies today:

> "The epileptic is avoided, on all faces he reads his sentence to isolation. Everywhere he goes, menacing and insurmountable obstacles arise to his obtaining a position, to establishing himself, to his relationships, and to his very livelihood; he has to say goodbye to his dreams of success, for the masters even refuse him work in their shops; goodbye to his dreams of marriage and fatherhood, goodbye to the joys of domestic hearth. This is death to the spirit."

7
1994

THE SUMMER AFTER freshman year, I was hired to help with an ongoing medical research project. My advisor was Thomas Jacoby, Ph.D., at the Medical College of Wisconsin in Milwaukee. Dr. Jacoby was a short, mysterious man with a staccato voice and harsh lines engraved in his face that belied his jovial demeanor. His shiny, bald head reflected ambient light and complimented his quick, bright smile. Dr. Jacoby researched the effect of simple verbal interventions with patients in a doctor's waiting room. He hoped to prove that short discussions with patients about positive lifestyle changes—like healthy eating, increasing exercise, or quitting smoking—could be done by trained personnel while patients waited for their physician. My job for the eight weeks between June and August 1994 was to sit in the waiting room of an urban Milwaukee clinic and offer patients a simple survey of four easy questions about their smoking history and willingness to quit smoking.

I learned a lot about medicine, and the human race in general, when I sat for hours in a family physician's waiting room. I carefully observed all cross-sections of society while I hid behind my wooden clipboard. Most memorable to me was a large family that stumbled in together early one weekday morning. The mother, clearly over-whelmed and in pain on crutches, watched her three rambunctious children touch and explore every aspect of the large room with weary eyes. They turned over books and newspapers and jumped on and off the furniture while she sat in the corner, fanning herself and rubbing her leg that was wrapped in a dirty bandage and propped on the nearest chair. She was the image of stress and exhaustion.

Next to her, a coifed middle-aged businessman tried unsuc-cessfully to build invisible walls around his pressed suit, leather briefcase, and crisp morning paper as he barely concealed his dis-dain for the rowdy scene. Another elderly lady averted her eyes and readjusted her earrings when the children threatened to come near.

Over that summer, I discovered that illness is a common denom-inator. Whether rich or poor, alone or ensconced with a gaggle of children, illness doesn't recognize socioeconomic status, intelligence, or ability to cope with a challenge. No matter how many walls we attempt to build around us, whether with a crutch or with a harsh stare, we return to level ground when we're vulnerable, exposed, or need to depend on others. Similarly, I could pretend I wasn't like those *other kids* with epilepsy, but I was in the same neurology office waiting room, petitioning for help and hoping for a cure.

I couldn't wait to be on the other side of the waiting room wall. My work that summer made me even more aware what a privi-lege it would be to provide care to children and families. I hoped to make a difference and touch lives. The clipboard and waiting room were miles away from my eventual goal, but they taught me to see patients beyond their diseases, whether they're ready to cope with illness or so overwhelmed by life that their needs are overlooked.

*   *   *

College was a blissful and carefree four years. Although my classes were rigorous and it felt like the material I needed to learn was endless, I loved learning about the science behind human interac-tions, the elemental building blocks of plants and animals, and the chemical composition of matter and species that constitute life. In addition to Jeff, Lisa, and Tim, my closest friends were the other students who worked at the library late into the night. Dark-haired and gregarious Sapna met me at the vending machines at 2 A.M. where we talked about our work and other stressors of the day. In my study cubicle, ebullient and bright-eyed Sue and I compared notes on the latest biology chapter and commiserated about upcoming exams. Overburdened yet soulful Sara tacked back and forth between whether pharmacy school or medical school was right for her. We were the self-proclaimed "library clique" from Monday through Thursday. On the weekends, my studious friends went to bars and parties and later told stories of their exciting outings. Instead, I drank coffee late into the evening with my other sober friends and wondered: was I missing something?

Still, I lived the same erratic life as my classmates. I went to bed at three in the morning, got up at nine, and ran around constantly in between. On the weekends, I allowed myself to sleep until noon. Coffee and persistent motion kept me functional, but I always felt like I was tempting the devil. Other than ignoring my need to sleep, I was a diligent patient and took my epilepsy medication as directed at the start and finish of each day. I methodically counted my pills at the end of each month and made the two-mile walk to the nearest Walgreen's on the Capitol Square for my refills.

During my early college years, epilepsy was both a distant memory and a constant presence. I hadn't had a seizure since my senior year of high school, and was completely acclimated to my medicine. At the same time, I lived in constant fear that everything could change in the space between breaths. I worried that I might have a seizure in my dorm room, the classroom, or on the crowded streets of downtown Madison. I was nowhere near as carefree as I wanted to be.

Eventually, though, like an insuppressible weed that has grown thick roots underground, epilepsy again sprouted to the surface. During my junior year, when I was overtired or emotionally stressed, a smattering of complex partial seizures returned. By the fall of my senior year, I was reliably having a small cluster of complex partial seizures each month immediately before my cycle. I tried my best to control things as well as I could, but I was both too busy to care and too worried to make changes. Afraid that changes in medication or new diagnostic tests could alter my blissful college life, I avoided mentioning the new seizures to anyone.

One frigid weekend afternoon during my junior year, my friend Jeff and I were eating lunch in the cafeteria next to our dorm. We cleared our weathered plastic trays and set the thin metal silverware in tubs to soak while we shared ideas for an upcoming assignment for our creative writing class.

"I think we should write about our experiences tutoring a group of at-risk kids in Madison," Jeff said.

"Now how could we do that?" I asked.

Were we going to flat-out invent this story? Jeff loved to pull my leg. His practical jokes—like the time he barricaded my roommate and me in our dorm room with used beer cans—were legendary in Sellery Hall.

"There's an after-school program called Project Jamaa that's run by the Madison Urban League. They would provide transportation to a local middle school once a week if we agreed to work with struggling students."

"Sounds great. How do we sign up?" We stepped outside into the freezing air. Icy snow crunched under our feet, and we hastened to cover every spare inch of exposed skin. I braved Wisconsin winters all my life and loved to watch the East coast newbies learn to do so.

Suddenly, beyond the commotion of buttoning coats and swirling scarves, a high-pitched cry rang out near the entrance to the cafeteria. We rushed along with the crowd and found my friend, Patricia, unconscious and seizing on the hard ground. Violent muscle spasms ripped open her thick coat as she convulsed. I stepped away in fear and watched a version of the very event I'd dreaded for the past several years.

Patricia's friend, a nursing student, knew first aid management for seizures. After she instructed a bystander to call 9-1-1, she rushed forward and placed a folded coat under Patricia's head to protect her from injury. Then she cleared any rocks, refuse, or sharp objects from the surrounding area to protect Patricia's quaking body from injury. She checked her watch and timed the seizure while she reassured the building crowd that our friend would be OK. She didn't make any attempt to hold her down to stop the convulsing and she avoided putting anything in Patricia's mouth. She knew that the antiquated fear that people who have epilepsy could swallow their tongue is false.

Minutes later, two kind men in black emergency medical uniforms covered Patricia in a blanket and loaded her gently onto a gurney after the seizure stopped. I stood with the pack of concerned students and watched while Patricia was loaded into the waiting ambulance. The sheer physical violence that resulted from a brainstorm of electrical activity was breathtaking. For the first time, I had a true appreciation of the intensity of epilepsy. I may have control of my actions, my choices, and my body most of the time, but when epilepsy appeared with its vitriol and vigor, I was also a helpless victim in the storm.

8
1995

FOR A FORMER church organist and choirgirl, the Lutheran Campus Center (LCC) was the ideal place to find a niche on the massive UW campus. I entered the drab, brown building with hesitancy and skepticism at first. Ensconced by the towering chemistry building on one side and an imposing Lutheran cathedral on the other, the LCC was easy to overlook. Its worn orange chairs and threadbare carpet seemed out of place in the vibrant college community. Since the building was built as a gathering place for Lutheran college students in the 1970s, the multiple study rooms, upstairs library overlooking campus, and even the larger multipurpose room were draped with variations of orange, green, and dark brown tapestries. It wasn't long, however, before I met the two people who infused life into the LCC far beyond its meager walls. Pastors Brent and Laurie welcomed me with enthusiasm, a warm meal, and even brought homemade cookies to my dorm room.

I returned to the LCC week after week and realized that the frayed spots on the orange chairs were patterned so after thousands of hours of use as students sat together talking, laughing, or studying. The massive stone hearth in the center of the entrance was a perfect spot to warm frozen hands and weary hearts. I quickly made friends with the other members of the LCC choir (which I joined, of course.) The humble building nestled in the shadows of campus formed the perfect respite for me.

I met a memorable new student in the choir early in my sophomore year. In fact, I heard Andrew before I saw him. He had a deep, bass voice that resonated across the rehearsal room into the hallway. When I walked up to the rehearsal room to join the group, Andrew's distinctive jocular laugh rang out.

When the singing stopped, we were introduced. Andrew's bright green eyes held mine until he noticed the hat I wore and circled closer. "Nice to meet you, Kristin. Is that an equation on your hat? Pi Beta...what's that Greek letter?" he asked the others with mounting sarcasm. "You're not in a *sorority*, are you?"

I went on the defensive. "It's Pi Beta Phi. I just joined recently but I'm nothing like most sorority girls!"

My decision to join the sorority was strongly encouraged by my mother and grandmother. I still wasn't sure how I'd fit in in a place where drinking parties were a prominent part of the culture.

Andrew sensed my unease but didn't back off. He added playfully, "A sorority! Am I even cool enough to talk to you?"

I shrank into the carpet and my friends giggled guiltily. I blinked back hot tears of frustration and embarrassment and completed the rest of the rehearsal with my eyes glued to the music. As soon as I was able, I slipped out of the room and slinked back to my dorm. I hated when people made assumptions about me based on my clothes, my looks, or a superfluous label on the back of my hat. I may've belonged to a sorority, but the real me was so much, much more.

I never wore my Pi Beta Phi sorority hat to the LCC again. Despite my initial impressions, I learned to appreciate Andrew's biting sense of humor and affection for teasing. His bass complimented my alto, and his extroverted nature contrasted nicely to my introverted core. Before long, a friendship grew.

*   *   *

During the winter of my senior year in college, I served as a practice pianist for the vocalists at the LCC while we prepared for a musical. One of the vocalists I worked with was Andrew. I began to appreciate the humor in his jokes as I stole short glimpses into his kind heart. When he suggested that we go skiing with another friend on a frigid Friday night, I jumped at the chance to sail through the winter air with friends.

Winter in Wisconsin is a season like no other. Most outsiders would curse the pervasive darkness and biting cold; for native Wisconsinites, however, winter is a season known for its bright white snowfalls, icy temperatures, and crystal clear days that are sparklingly beautiful and pure. Wisconsin winter landscapes washed with snow and ice are a kind of unique perfection.

True, dressing for the outdoors—in my case, a coat, snow pants, boots, gloves, hat, long underwear, regular underwear, and ear warmers—could take the romance out of a setting. But when I stood in the middle of a snowfall, looked up into the mottled depth of sky and felt the stillness of the muffled silence that came with a storm, I was reminded why I lived in the Upper Midwest.

On the evening of our ski date, Andrew, our friend Jeremy, and I pulled up to Cascade Mountain just after 4:00, as the sun slipped behind the distant hills and the interminable darkness crept in. We put on our gear while the remaining pale light in the sky drained away. The horizon shifted from purple to black. Soon the electric hum of the surrounding overhead lights grew and the hills were illuminated with an unnatural florescent brightness. The ski lift carried us up the mountain and back in time. I felt like a giddy child when we careened down the hill and my worries flew away in the powder and mist. With each run down the hill, the carefully constructed protective layers built to guard my emotions weakened a bit more. We sat on the chair lift with our hanging skis dripping hijacked snow back to the distant ground and laughed so hard that the tears froze to our cheeks and the smiles froze to our faces. Winter didn't get any better than this.

When Andrew helped me off the lift before one of the last runs of the evening, I tripped and almost fell before his padded coat and gloved hands caught me. For an instant, he held me next to his warm body as if it were the most natural thing in the world. He paused for only a moment before I was pushed playfully downhill. I regained my bearings before I put my skis in parallel position and pushed snow to the right, then the left and worked my way down the hill. We rode home in the comfort and warmth of the car while we sipped hot chocolate and enjoyed each other's company. It wasn't long before my mind confirmed what my heart already knew.

*   *   *

E

Early historical treatments for epilepsy varied depending on the beliefs about seizures at the time. Before Hippocrates, when epilepsy was thought to be due to a curse or possession by evil spirits, patients would offer sacrifices or take part in religious acts under supervision of a "doctor-priest."

In 400 BC, Hippocrates wrote the classic text **On the Sacred Disease**, which included some of the earliest records of epilepsy in humans. He was one of the first people to assert that epilepsy has a natural cause and he advocated treating the disease with natural means.[6] Hippocrates, however, believed that seizures are caused by too much phlegm on the brain and his treatments focused on a restrictive diet, regulation of excretions, and physiotherapy. He went as far as recommending a craniotomy on the opposite side of the brain to relieve patients of the build-up of phlegm that caused their disease. Herbs and early medicines took a secondary role.

As supporters of Hippocratic medicine dwindled between the 1st and 6th centuries, a single theologian and several medical experts recommended the consumption of the blood or liver of a slain gladiator to cure epilepsy. The ban on gladiatorial combat in 400 AD led physicians to endorse the ingestion of the blood of an executed individual, especially if he were beheaded.[7] Despite Hippocrates' assertions, by the Middle Ages epilepsy was again thought to have a religious origin and therapy returned to the use of sacred objects or saints to intercede with God on their behalf.

Finally, during the 1920s, a German psychiatrist named Hans Berger developed the human electroencephalograph (EEG). The EEG recorded and revealed the electrical patterns of brainwaves and definitively showed the abnormal electrical discharges associated with seizures. The EEG also helped locate the origin of atypical discharges and provided the framework for later neurosurgical treatments for epilepsy. With the electrographic evidence that seizures have an origin within the electrical framework of the brain, treatments focused on finding medications that could tame the aberrant electrical activity instead of trying to rid the body of demons or curses. One hundred years later, however, treatment for seizures and public acceptance of epilepsy continues to evolve.

9
1996

AFTER A HANDFUL of "non-dates" when we went to dinner to discuss friendship and the treble clef, Andrew and I finally acknowledged our affection for each other the following spring. Once we were officially dating, trips to the coffee shop or even the grocery store became moments of wonder as we learned about our mutual interests and desires and fell deeply in love. Some of my previous relationships had ended because I was unwilling to reveal my fragile inner self. This time, with Andrew, things were almost immediately different.

I confessed my most private hopes and dreams and my most ominous worries and fears. I didn't have to tell Andrew about my epilepsy because somehow he already knew. Most of my college comrades knew I didn't drink alcohol because of a vague medical reason. When the LCC choir went on overnight road trips, Andrew noticed that I was the only person in the group who carried "a bunch of medications." When it was time to tell him my full story, I downplayed the shadow that epilepsy cast on my everyday life. It was years before both Andrew and I understood that the threat of seizures would be a constant in our relationship and that uncertainty would be a common denominator for all of our days.

In fact, epilepsy was one reason why I tried to precisely control all other aspects of my life. Since the day in high school when my brother Jon showed me his gross anatomy cadaver, I knew the professional path I would follow and I meticulously planned every step along the way. Each apartment I ever lived in was unique for its orderliness and neatness. This aspect of my personality drove my family crazy but it comforted me. I'd been surprised by seizures in the middle of the day, when falling asleep at night, in the middle of classrooms, or while doing mundane things like washing my hands or drying my hair. It didn't come unexpected, then, that my need to create order in other parts of my life partially offset the chaos of sudden seizures. Andrew accepted this part of me early on, and for that, I'm grateful.

On a summer afternoon after we began dating, Andrew and I rode our bikes through the sunshine along the rugged shore of Lake Mendota. We ogled houses by the lake, rode past rows of offices and shops, and finally took a break from biking at a verdant park on the north shoreline. We walked our bikes to a natural patch of shore and enjoyed the view of the Capitol and campus across the water. Andrew sat on a boulder next to the water and beckoned me to sit next to him. For a while, we listened to the rhythmic *pssh pssh pssh* of the waves as they gently crashed into the rocks.

Andrew turned and kissed me while his arm warmed my shoulder. "You know, this is going to sound crazy," he said, his green eyes swimming in the silent heat, "but I think I love you."

I studied Andrew's face and felt an energy and excitement I'd never known. I finally understood what love was. Tentatively, I spoke, "I think I love you, too." The protective walls around my heart crashed down, and I turned to meet his lips.

With this confession, we embarked on the partnership that would last the rest of our lives.

*   *   *

My seizures increased in strength and frequency during the same spring I fell in love. I found a new neurologist in Madison since my schedule made it increasingly hard to make regular trips to Milwaukee to follow-up with my previous neurologist. It wasn't hard to find a physician who specialized in the care of patients with epilepsy in a town with a nationally known academic medical center.

The adult neurology clinic was hidden deep in the catacombs of the University of Wisconsin hospital. I passed several different waiting rooms full of anxious people nervously awaiting the unknown as I walked through the winding hospital corridors. Original pictures of local wildlife dotted the final grey hall that led to the neurology and urology suites. I admired a photograph of a butterfly resting on a flower, another of tall grass bending in the wind in the Class of 1918 Marsh. The pictures were a refreshing reminder of life and beauty in a seemingly endless hallway of expectation.

A familiar, distinct smell filled the air just before I reached my destination. The saccharine sweetness of the glue that technicians use to attach EEG electrodes to a patient's head was as familiar to me as my own reflection. The unmistakable odor, potent in its sweetness and acidity, immediately conjured memories of my hospitalization and diagnosis of epilepsy just a few years before.

I approached the check-in desk adorned with thick block letters exclaiming ADULT NEUROLOGY. I announced my presence and the receptionist directed me to take a seat. I settled in, scanned the room, and remembered my summer experience in a waiting room where I observed patients who could've been me.

Before long, an assistant called my name and I was brought back to a small exam room.

"What brings you here?" The kind medical assistant wore a badge with "Cheryl B" written on it, the last part of her name blocked with white tape. Cheryl eyed me inquisitively while she measured my pulse, blood pressure, and other vital signs.

"I have epilepsy." Admitting it to someone else sounded so certain, so final. I continued to wish that epilepsy were a thing of the past, although I was reminded of my illness whenever I had a cluster of seizures each month.

"When was your last seizure?" she asked.

I was so used to hiding my seizures that it was difficult to answer.

"I had two little seizures three weeks ago," I admitted. I expected surprise or a question when Cheryl jotted notes in my chart, but there were none.

"Dr. Rodgers will be right in." Cheryl flipped the chart closed and whirled out of the exam room door.

A gentle knock on the door followed shortly thereafter. Dr. Rodgers was a tall, thin man in his mid-forties. He had a kind smile and silver hair that complimented his white coat. His firm handshake confirmed his confidence and knowledge. He stretched behind the desk with the thin file created by Cheryl B and glanced at the few notes written.

"So you have epilepsy. Tell me your story." He leaned forward expectantly to listen. Words came tumbling out so quickly that I wasn't sure they made sense.

A weight slowly lifted as I rambled through the history of my first prolonged seizure and subsequent smaller, monthly seizures. The veil shrouding this portion of my life had become so opaque that only a closed, tight circle knew.

Dr. Rodgers nodded and grunted affirmation. When I finished, his lips curved into a small crescent smile and his eyes held mine.

"You're going to think I'm crazy," he ventured, "but I think you're a candidate for surgery."

I was so shocked, I couldn't respond or even process the idea of brain surgery before he continued.

"Based on your description of your seizures and the history of prolonged febrile seizure in early childhood, I believe you have temporal lobe epilepsy."

The room around us began to fall away, and Dr. Rodgers' voice became crisp and precise, like a hammer pounding nails in the coffin of my carefree life. I imagined myself sitting alone on a stage with a spotlight glaring down. Above me flashed large, white signs that read DAMAGED and DISEASED. Friends, mentors, and acquaintances packed the audience of my reverie. I imagined their confusion and consternation when the self-induced secret of my epilepsy was disclosed.

The labels I'd shed in the past but could never completely abandon danced with menacing threats to my confidence and independence.

Dr. Rodgers explained that temporal lobe seizures are notoriously the hardest to control. "We don't have many medications in our arsenal that are 100% effective in controlling temporal lobe epilepsy. Each patient is different, but surgical removal of the seizure focus—in your case, your temporal lobe—is often the best hope to achieve a cure."

"Where is my temporal lobe?" I asked.

"Your temporal lobes are roughly above your ears on both sides of your head. The vascular and energy supply to the deepest parts of the temporal lobe, structures called the hippocampus and amygdala, are some of the first parts of your brain to suffer if you have a prolonged seizure. Any portion of the human brain that is deprived of its vital flow of oxygen and nutrients can suffer irreparable damage. I believe that you have a small damaged area in your temporal lobe that's now the focal point of your seizures."

"What do those structures you talked about do?" As a college senior, I was woefully unfamiliar with my medical terminology.

"The hippocampus is the area of the brain that stores short-term memory." I sensed Dr. Rodgers' excitement as he talked about his area of expertise. "I think your hippocampus is involved in your seizures because of the sensation of déjà vu you have at the beginning of your seizures."

I was flabbergasted by this observation. The feeling of déjà vu had become so bothersome to me over time that I became fearful of an oncoming seizure whenever a conversation or event triggered a memory. Imagine that there was an actual anatomic basis for my fears.

Dr. Rodgers continued, "The amygdala drives sensations like fear and panic. It also converts short-term memory to long-term memory and regulates our emotional reactions to memories."

Another light bulb went off. The discomfort in my abdomen that my childhood pediatrician diagnosed as reflux was more adequately described to others as the sensation of "butterflies in the stomach." It was the same feeling I had when I was playing piano for a crowd, performing in a play, or taking an important exam. Since this sensation occurred prior to each one of my seizures, I'd wondered if there was a component of nervousness or anxiety that triggered my episodes. Dr. Rodgers' explanation that abnormal electrical activity in the amygdala could produce these visceral reactions was enlightening.

Dr. Rodgers ordered an MRI of my brain to confirm his suspicion. He predicted the MRI would reveal temporal lobe scarring, or sclerosis. He also arranged for a Positive Emission Tomography (PET) scan to determine if the area in question had the same or lesser amounts of normal activity than the other areas of my brain. Dr. Rodgers explained that a PET scan is a specialized radiology procedure that uses a small amount of a radioactive tracer to evaluate the metabolism of a specific organ or tissue. He expected that there were areas in my temporal lobe that were less functional than the rest of my brain. The results of these tests would guide the long-term management of my seizures.

Dr. Rodgers finished the visit by stating that if the diagnostic tests helped define the focus of my seizures, surgery to remove the affected part of my brain may offer a 95% chance of reduction in seizures or, perhaps, even a *cure* for epilepsy.

I walked out of my first appointment at the adult neurology clinic with mixed emotions. Mostly, I was excited. Since diagnosed with epilepsy, I'd assumed that I would always live with medications and seizures. The prospect of finding a cure for my illness represented a paradigm shift. I would no longer focus on how to live well with epilepsy, but instead how I could achieve living without it.

At the same time, I was terrified. The idea of starting a series of specialized tests and considering brain surgery while simultaneously studying to become a physician seemed impossible. And, of course, what if I had the surgery—putting my career and life at risk—only to find that I was one of the 5% of patients who didn't improve or find a cure?

I tried to explain my emotions to the polished linoleum floors with my head cast down, hair shrouding my face, and tears welling in my eyes. I felt hopeful and encouraged, yet wary and scared. Above all, I felt alone.

* * *

E

The history of epilepsy surgery began as early as 1909, when Harvey Cushing reported sensory responses and sensory auras that were similar to focal seizures produced by electrical simulation in two patients awake under local anesthesia.[8] By 1912, neurosurgeon Fedor Krause was able to draw a detailed map of the human brain after he carefully observed muscular contractions of the face and extremities while he stimulated different areas of a patient's brain. Over time, careful monitoring of a patient's symptoms or seizure type led physicians to determine which part of the brain was involved in seizures.

Seizures arising in the temporal lobe became a subject of increasing interest from 1945–1955. Until that time, surgery was directed mostly at abnormalities on the outer surface of the brain and most often for removal of tumors or traumatic scars. Neurosurgeons first recommended that patients with temporal lobe epilepsy have a small portion of their temporal lobe removed to avoid complications. The first series of patients who had this operation had a success rate of just over 50%. As the surgery was refined and improved, the surgical success rate increased to up to 80% by 1991, and the anterior temporal lobectomy became the gold standard of care for treatment of patients with medically intractable temporal lobe seizures.[9]

10
1997

I RECEIVED MY undergraduate degree from the University of Wisconsin in the spring of 1997, shortly after my first and fateful visit with Dr. Rodgers. I spent the following summer working at a Madison coffee shop and enjoying long afternoons with Andrew. I also completed my MRI, PET scan, and another EEG as recommended by Dr. Rodgers. I nervously awaited the next neurology visit while I prepared to embark in the next major phase of my education.

The University of Wisconsin Medical School held a White Coat Ceremony to welcome incoming first year students to medical school. Proud parents, dear friends, and exhilarated new students anxiously awaited the traditional event each year. The faculty at the white coat ceremony marked our official entry into physician training by sheathing each new student with a pristine white coat adorned with the UW crest. Many tears were shed as my 155 classmates and I marched into the auditorium at the Memorial Union to participate in the ceremony. The lights were dimmed so we couldn't see the crowd of friends, family, and supporters behind us. A bright red banner stretched across the front stage stated simply: "Welcome University of Wisconsin Medical School Class of 2001!"

I took my seat and heaved a sigh of relief as I settled in.

Finally.

Years of anticipation, expectation, and hard work paved the path to this auditorium. I shared the stage and the moment with some of the brightest young minds from all over the country, all of us singly focused on a dream. A chill ran down my spine.

The keynote speaker reminded us to work hard, nurture empathy and compassion, and to take time to learn the "art" of medicine. My classmates smiled together when the Dean stood before us and asked us to recite the Medical Student Oath:

> As I enter the medical profession,
>
> I will remember that I am a member of a larger community, with social responsibility to all, both sick and well.
>
> I will respect the efforts of my teachers and colleagues, and I will not hesitate to ask for their assistance when needed.
>
> I will not let gender, race, sexual preference, or religion prejudice my interactions with patients or colleagues.
>
> I will protect the privacy of my patients, and I will keep my interactions with them confidential.
>
> I will remember that medicine is a multifaceted discipline, combining art and science, with the aim of preventing disease when possible, treating when necessary, and above all expressing genuine empathy and understanding to patients and families.
>
> I will remember that in order to properly care for my patients, I must also take care of myself, both body and spirit.

One by one, the Dean called us to the stage to put on our white coats. When it was my turn, I was surprised that the thick, crisp sleeves of the white coat made me feel restricted. I percolated with burgeoning altruism and ambition yet the unforgiving white coat hindered me. Eventually I would learn that medicine, like the coat, did not give. The White Coat Ceremony marked my entry into a profession that would never allow for compromise or "just enough." I viewed the future and saw tears, academic pressure, endless nights, the loss of my youth, and challenges to my health, all for the distinction of wearing a white coat.

Later, I wrote the last line of the Medical Student Oath on a piece of thick paper and tacked it to my bulletin board. Even as the paper yellowed, the quote stayed fixed within view and traveled with me from apartment to apartment throughout medical school and into my residency training. The simple phrase helped me remember to take a breath and—at least temporarily—try to meet my own needs. Over time, I learned that the human body can last a long time while deprived of regular sleep, vacation, or time to relax. The human spirit, however, involutes when neglected and leaves only a cold, cynical shell which functions proficiently yet mindlessly. Ever since my first day of medical school, I have fought to maintain the essence of what drew me toward medicine, a love affair that has always burned bright.

*   *   *

After my initial discussion with Dr. Rodgers about potential brain surgery, my family invited themselves to my next neurology appointment. In the months between my first and second visit to U.W. Neurology Clinic, the dual existence of life as both a medical professional and a patient emerged. By day, I was an eager first year medical student who tried my best to absorb the mass of material in my textbooks, anatomy drawings, and lab sessions. In the evenings, I was a patient with epilepsy. I tentatively navigated the foreign paths that led to more diagnostic tests and procedures and attempted to ward off the threatening seizures that often woke me at night.

When I walked with my family, the long, brick hallway that led to the neurology suite didn't seem quite so ominous. My mother, father, Andrew, and my brother, Jon, surrounded me in a protective circle. Jon enjoyed his new role as a surgical resident at the

University of Wisconsin. I occasionally ran into him, scrub-clad and weary-eyed, when I took classes at the hospital.

Jon picked up many of our father's mannerisms as a young boy. He and Dad both subtly portrayed their softness and affection by their actions and presence instead of with words. Jon especially had a sympathetic heart. He came to my appointment still in his worn scrubs and mentioned only when asked that he'd been operating for the past eight hours. I was comforted by his knowledge of the medical field. He asked many questions in medical jargon and helped interpret Dr. Rodgers' impressions and recommendations in a way that we all could understand.

We crammed into the small exam room in the neurology office and waited. You could almost hear our collective nervous energy buzzing in the room. My parents asked Jon about his latest surgical rotation and Andrew's hand rubbed my knee. We pretended we were enjoying a typical family gathering.

Eventually, Dr. Rodgers arrived and seated himself in the only vacant chair in the small space. The manila folder that housed my medical records had grown significantly thicker since my previous visit.

"Well," Dr. Rodgers began, "I'm glad to see all of you here to talk about the best treatment for Kristin's epilepsy." He reviewed the results of the recently performed diagnostic tests.

"Your MRI confirms that you have a small area of scarring in your right hippocampus. Neurologists refer to this as hippocampal sclerosis, which is one of the most common causes of temporal lobe epilepsy."

My parents were confused by the medical terminology; Jon and I leaned in to hear more.

"Your PET scan also shows decreased metabolism—or decreased overall function—in your right temporal lobe. While this is atypical in patients without a history of seizures, this confirms that your prolonged seizure as a toddler left its mark. This also corroborates the diagnosis of temporal lobe epilepsy."

While Dr. Rodgers talked, he hung the images from the PET scan and MRI on a light box on the wall. Though small, I found the scarred area that shone with more radioactive tracer on the left than its mirror image on the right.

My mom asked the question forming on my lips. "How can Kristin function so normally if there is a whole section of her brain that is damaged and scarred?"

"The human brain is remarkable for its plasticity. When a traumatic event happens early in life, the brain has the ability to form new electrical connections that eventually eliminate the need for the injured area at all."

Dr. Rodgers continued, "I believe that the majority of Kristin's right temporal lobe has little beneficial function but harbors the focus of her seizures. The identical structures on the left side of her brain are enough for Kristin to maintain normal cognitive ability and function."

We took a moment to digest this information before Dad spoke. "The surgery you proposed—what would that involve?"

Dr. Rodgers explained that removing the seizure focus in my right temporal lobe might be my best chance at achieving freedom from seizures. It sounded so simple, yet so terrifying.

I continued to listen, mesmerized, as Dr. Rodgers explained what surgery would entail.

"During the surgery, called a temporal lobectomy, a neurosurgeon would remove a portion of your brain about the size of a lime." He made a shape between his thumb and forefinger that represented the size of a lime but instead looked like a broken 'A-Okay' signal to me. "Because Kristin's seizure focus is on the right side of her brain and she is right-handed, the left, or dominant side, of her brain most likely holds her executive speech function. We would confirm this prior to surgery, but I would expect that removal of Kristin's right temporal lobe would not affect her speech and language capabilities. Similarly, because I don't think Kristin has used her right temporal lobe for memory or cognitive tasks since she was a toddler, extraction of this area should have no bearing on her ability to become a physician. Because the temporal lobe does not guide any motor tasks, her physical movement and activities should not be affected."

Dr. Rodgers took a breath and continued. "However, the nerves that carry electrical messages from the left upper quarter of her visual field would be severed during a right temporal lobectomy. After the surgery, patients are left with a left upper quadrant visual field defect. Over time, this defect is largely unnoticed because only a small portion of peripheral vision is gone. As with any major neurosurgical procedure, there would be a small risk of stroke and a small risk of infection.

"Though your preliminary testing and history appear favorable, there is no guarantee that surgery will render a cure for your epilepsy... however, this may be your best chance to improve or eliminate your seizures."

Since the prospect of brain surgery was formidable, my parents suggested that we speak to another neurologist for a second opinion. Dr. Rodgers referred us to a colleague at Mayo Clinic. I sat in the corner of the room and tried to make sense of my conflicting emotions while my parents talked more with Dr. Rodgers. As a first year medical student, I was intrigued by his explanations of a brain's plasticity, right temporal lobe function, and how a lime-sized piece of my brain could be removed with few untoward effects. As a patient, my mind swam with thoughts of visual field defects, infection, stroke, or possibly a cure for epilepsy. My newly acquired professional rational impulses conflicted with my deeply ingrained emotional fragility. Only months into my formal medical training, I'd already learned that when an anatomical problem is found, it's best to take the quickest steps to fix it. In the same amount of time, I forgot to consider the toll that this could take.

My brother's wife, Beth, joined us for lunch at The Olive Garden after the appointment. My family talked animatedly about the weather, the Badgers' football season, and Jon's residency. With the help of breadsticks, salad, and lively conversation, we effectively and deliberately avoided the elephant in the room as well as the feelings uprooted and implications made from my appointment. I chose to cope with my swimming thoughts of seizures, brain surgery, and uncertainty in the same way I'd learned to manage other things that worry me: ignore and move on.

My parents and boyfriend talked and laughed together as I sat in silence and idly pushed the food around on my plate. Part of me no longer felt a part of their easy lives; instead, I felt as if I was observing them from behind a window outside. I sighed and dove into my salad. The food filled the empty place in my gut carved out by fear. Ignore and move on. Ignore and move on.

I resolved to move past my anxiety and re-join the present. After all, there was too much to do. Epilepsy wasn't part of my plan.

11

THE FIRST AND SECOND year medical students at the University of Wisconsin ran a group of free clinics in Madison called the MEDIC clinics. All students were encouraged to volunteer as providers in the clinics once or twice a semester. When the opportunity arose, I signed the MEDIC volunteer sheet immediately. I was eager to learn things outside of my esoteric anatomy and physiology classes and couldn't wait for the chance to provide actual patient care.

I walked to my first assignment at the Salvation Army MEDIC clinic on a grey fall afternoon. The warmth of summer had given way quickly to a creeping cold breeze that warned of another winter to come. I admired the remnants of the passing season as I ambled down East Washington Avenue. Crimson oak leaves rested in velvet piles next to golden birch and orange maple leaves in a low-lying autumn rainbow. While I waited at a stoplight, a puff of wind blew across the crosswalk and created a fleeting tornado of leaves that quickly dissolved a few feet away.

Eventually, I walked up to a squat building with block letters across the top that read S LV TION RMY. The outer walls of the building were marred with dirt streaks and scars. Several men played basketball in a corner of the parking lot. They threw the bright orange ball to each other and toward the bare hoop attached to the backboard by a single metal wire. My protected suburban upbringing offered little exposure to the inner city landscape. I didn't know what to expect at the Salvation Army.

I shuffled quickly into the building. Bright lights, bouncing balls, and the sounds of children playing in the gym met me. I wandered down the hall and found my way to a bare conference room where two of my classmates sat at a worn oak table. We exchanged nervous glances and I settled in.

Dr. Krall was the physician director of the Salvation Army MEDIC clinic. He ambled into the room with his well-fed belly leading the way. He had an unruly grey beard, bushy eyebrows that looked like floating puffs of clouds, and eyes that exuded kindness and empathy. Dr. Krall addressed us in a formal, businesslike manner.

"Welcome to the Salvation Army. Tonight, you will provide care to children and families at a time when they are most vulnerable. The residents of the Salvation Army are single women with dependent children in need of a safe place to stay. Each family can remain here for up to ninety days at a time. All of our residents receive three meals a day and an evening snack along with adult education classes on life skills, employment, and parenting. We have capacity for up to eighteen families at a time."

Dr. Krall took a slow, purposeful breath before he spoke again. He looked deliberately from student to student, daring each of us to rise to his challenge.

"Try to reserve your judgment of these women and children. Ask them to tell you how they came to live here and you will be surprised by what you hear. Many of the women work one or two jobs but do not earn enough to pay for safe housing. Others have tales of tragedy, hardship, or circumstances beyond their control. You'll be astounded by their stories."

Dr. Krall again eyed us one by one. I shrank in my chair when his gaze fell upon me, embarrassed by my preconceived notions and belief that I was somehow better than the families who lived at the Salvation Army. I simply was luckier.

I sat, reflected, and recognized that every life has its own challenges. My brother had asthma, my school friend had cancer, and my classmate from high school lost her father at an early age. My friend had a brother with Down syndrome, my neighbor struggled in school, I had epilepsy.

In many ways, epilepsy made me more human. When I was stricken with my illness as a toddler or with the grand mal seizure in high school, I was completely dependent on others. In a few important ways, I shared common ground with the women at the Salvation Army. I knew what helpless felt like. I'd experienced frustration to the point of despair from something beyond my control. I was anxious to do my small part to throw others a lifeline.

I had time to meet with only one family during my first night at MEDIC: a proud, handsome mother with three small children. The children all suffered from the runny nose and cough that were common in the community at the time. I used my limited first-year-medical-student-skills to listen to their lungs, look in their ears, and check their eyes. I noted the threadbare clothes that hung loosely on their bodies and their worn, dilapidated shoes when I quietly listened to each child in turn. Contrary to their attire, the children all had beautiful, broad smiles and bright, intelligent eyes.

The children's mother was disappointed when we diagnosed all three with viral colds that would take a week or more to resolve. She hoped for a quicker fix so she could return to work instead of staying home to care for her sick children. She accepted the offered samples of Tylenol and nasal saline quietly and plunged the bottles deep into her purse for safekeeping. When the visit ended, I gave each child a free book from the local Reach Out and Read program. Their faces lit with joy when they held the books tightly to their grimy chests.

During the following hour, I examined a baby with an ear infection and an adolescent who jammed his finger while playing basketball. Later that evening, I found the woman with the three children sitting near the gymnasium in the middle of the hallway. The lines in her face carved by adversity were turned upward in a

gentle smile. She sat nestled against the wall with her children drap-
ing her sides and lap. Tenderly, she enclosed each of their shoulders
and arms in a wide embrace. The youngest child sat in the middle
of the family circle and held her brand new book high. Her mother
haltingly read the simple children's story in a singsong voice. They
were the image of fleeting contentment.

That night at the Salvation Army was the first time I recognized
that sometimes the best medicine has nothing to do with diagnosis, medications, or cure. At times, a simple gesture to temporarily
remove hardship or suffering can be the most potent medicine of all.

12

IT TOOK SEVERAL MONTHS to schedule a neurology appointment at Mayo Clinic. Finally, my mom and I travelled to Mayo the following summer to confirm that I might be a good candidate for epilepsy surgery. My parents and I never acknowledged our unspoken hope that if I visited as many specialists as possible, somehow I'd be safe. We drove for hours over picturesque bluffs, unmarred except for the linear asphalt scar that ran like a cord of black licorice through the countryside. My mother drove with methodical precision. Her eyes never deviated from the road, her hands remained firmly placed at the ten and two o'clock positions, and she was oblivious to the parade of cars that passed while she eked along at a steady fifty mph. The hours on the road with Mom were reminiscent of the long hours we travelled in our faux-wood station wagon on spring break as children. Whether headed for vacations or family visits to Florida or Montana, Indiana or Missouri, we always had fun. This trip, of course, was a little different.

We rolled into Rochester, Minnesota as the sun began its descent. We expected to find a busy urban center in the middle of the midwestern town home to the Mayo Clinic. Instead, we exited the highway onto a tree-lined street with charming well-kept houses and, occasionally, the quintessential picket fence. Scattered residents walked outside along the flawless white sidewalks. It seemed that the whole town subscribed to a pledge of calm.

We explored the area before heading downtown to check into our hotel. After a long day of driving, we were ready to relax and decompress. The manicured hotel clerk stood guard at the reception desk and welcomed us warmly. Mom asked if the hotel provided transportation for its guests to Mayo Clinic. The clerk's expression quickly changed from business-like to empathetic.

"Yes, of course we do. Our first shuttle leaves at 8:00 A.M. Will your daughter be accompanying you?"

We both felt obligated to correct the stranger's mistake. "Oh, she's the one with an appointment tomorrow," my mother pointed to me. "I'm here with her."

The clerk's eyes wandered to me and looked up and down slowly, no doubt wondering where the illness was hidden beneath my otherwise normal appearance. I pretended not to notice the scrutiny. Instead, I smiled brightly and spoke through my discomfort. "Do you have a pool?"

My mom and I resumed pretending our trip was no different than previous family vacations while the clerk explained the hotel's amenities. Despite the circumstances, I was glad to be on this trip with her. It was an opportunity to spend needed time together and strengthen the mother-daughter bond that'd weakened since I left for college. At the same time, however, I was profoundly uncomfortable. What would we gain from our trip to Mayo? Would the doctors here have anything different to say than my doctors in Madison? Would they recommend immediate hospital admission to begin a pre-surgical evaluation? Would they suggest different medications? Did they hold the key to my cure?

We awoke the following morning to birds chirping outside our window and air scented with the mid-summer blooms of lily and lilac. The dew lifted from the grass as the sun warmed the earth. I dressed quickly while Mom scoured the hotel information packet to find a place for breakfast. The lurking disquiet kept its distance when we concentrated on the basic tasks at hand.

After a quick breakfast, we were officially on our way. Mayo Clinic is a cluster of tall, foreboding office buildings that are home to some of the most talented medical specialists in the world. The outside view of the main building looked surprisingly similar to my college dormitory; an ominous, rectangular concrete structure striped with thin, geometric rows of windows encircling the building to the very top. A bronze statue of the two Mayo brothers sits comfortably on the front steps where they can observe the approaching clientele.

For a moment, my nervousness was overpowered by my awe of the mecca of modern medicine. Even during my first year of medical school, I learned about countless therapeutic discoveries born at Mayo and studied the work of physicians who practiced here. When we stepped inside, the sea of men and women dressed in dark blue blazers crisscrossing the main plaza impressed me. Mayo Clinic requires uniform dress so patients can easily identify the medical professionals. I wondered if the formal attire somehow made the doctors smarter or if it only made the patients more intimidated.

The neurologist I visited, Dr. Chad Shan, wore his dark blazer comfortably and greeted us warmly as he ushered us into office. The room had the unlikely appearance of a coffee shop. There was a stiff couch in the center of the room with several thick, plush chairs pushed against the walls and two mahogany end tables sparsely scattered with magazines. The far wall was lined with diplomas and certificates, evidence of his credibility and expertise. Dr. Shan settled himself in a leather chair at a small desk and invited Mom and me to sit across from him on the couch.

Dr. Shan listened to my medical history with meticulous attention and took copious notes as I spoke. He rustled through the stack of papers from Dr. Rodgers' office and scratched additional notes with a gleaming Cross fountain pen. I wondered if he might find a previously elusive answer in the inkblots of my medical history. He grunted and nodded while Mom talked but only occasionally lifted his piecing grey eyes to meet mine.

From my seat in the corner, I studied his diplomas and certificates one by one. There was his college diploma, a medical school graduation certificate, his framed state license and his residency graduation certificate. A plaque from his specialty fellowship training was most prominently displayed. My own professional goals weren't that different from what Dr. Shan had achieved. I wondered if epilepsy would prevent me from one day having a stack of diplomas of my own.

Dr. Shan turned his attention to me after Mom finished talking. "I understand you're in medical school, Kristin."

"Yes. I just completed my first year." I was proud to have one of the hardest years of medical school behind me.

He studied his notes. "Has it been hard to complete your studies with ongoing seizures?"

"A little bit, but I don't let them slow me down. Every now and then, I have to take a break if I have a seizure after a late-night study session. For the most part, I do okay." I paused and took a breath. "The fear of seizures is sometimes more bothersome than the seizures themselves. I'm more careful when I'm overtired, stressed, or if it's a certain time of the month because I know that I'm more prone to seizures then. Still, I never truly know when a seizure is going to change the course of an entire day.

"Mostly, I wish I could be free of that constant worry. I feel like I'm always walking on eggshells, waiting for one to crack." I swallowed back tears as I spoke. Dr. Shan's expression was compassionate.

Dr. Shan recommended that we repeat all of my previous diagnostic studies so he could collect his own data. He explained that the diagnostic imaging he was ordering used different radiographic techniques that may find other subtle abnormalities in my brain. He ordered a MRI, EEG, carbamazepine blood level, and PET scan. I quickly fell back into the patient role as I was ushered from one suite to the next over the following four days. My mom and I enjoyed more one-on-one time than we'd had in years. We giggled as we tricked doctor after doctor into thinking that *she* was the patient. One night we dined at an upscale Italian restaurant and pretended that we were simply enjoying a restful vacation together. Finally, after four days of testing, it was time to meet with Dr. Shan again.

Things were a little different when we returned to Dr. Shan's office for the second time that week. This time, Mom and I nervously awaited his arrival while seated together on the stiff, grey couch. I imagined being swept up immediately and admitted to the hospital for inpatient EEG monitoring. I was ready to move toward the end of my epilepsy—if it existed. Surgery seemed like the closest thing to a definite answer in my so-far journey of *maybe* and *we'll see*.

A single issue of *Reader's Digest* rested on the end table next to one of the enormous purple chairs. Mom read it cover to cover while we waited. I sat in silent anticipation as the minutes ticked by. After almost a week of companionable mother-daughter lunches, outings, and exploration, we were trapped in the hush of the consultation room. We sat for three solid hours and waited for Dr. Shan to appear, unmoving and rarely talking while cloaked with a cloud of uncertainty.

Finally, we heard a quiet knock on the door and Dr. Shan appeared. He brought no apology for his extreme tardiness, as if the Mayo blazer and credentials on the wall made it permissible. But he didn't waste any time once he sat in his familiar chair.

"I've had a chance to review your studies, Kristin, and it appears you definitely have temporal lobe epilepsy with a right temporal lobe focus." Dr. Shan was proud of this affirmation. I didn't know that there was ever any question.

He tacked a series of pictures from my most recent MRI on the light board in his office. Dr. Shan's fingers found the snail-like structure in the middle part of my brain that I now knew to be my hippocampus. He used his elegant fountain pen to point as he talked. "This is your hippocampus, where we believe short-term memory is stored. The hippocampus on the left side of your brain appears normal and healthy." He pointed to the same structure in the series of films. It was amazing how such a small collection of neurons could store vast volumes of data.

"If you turn your attention to the hippocampus on the right," Dr. Shan paused for effect, "you'll notice that the comparable region here looks bright white, small, and shriveled."

I remembered seeing a similar image of my hippocampus in Madison, but the pictures at Mayo were even more striking. My right hippocampus appeared like a dried worm on a scorched summer pavement instead of a normal, meaty, gently coiled snail.

Dr. Shan pointed emphatically to my shriveled worm and exclaimed, with a glint of excitement and discovery, "This little damaged region is the cause of your seizures."

He continued, "Your EEG was normal, but a one-hour EEG is like taking a quick picture of your brain waves when what we really need is a continuous recording to capture a seizure."

I was still picking the tacky EEG glue out of my hair and off my head even though the study was completed two days ago.

"Your blood test indicates that the amount of carbamazepine circulating in your bloodstream remains at a level within our goal range. Usually, patients who respond positively to carbamazepine are able to maintain seizure control or achieve a notable reduction in seizures at these levels."

Mom and I looked at each other. "So, putting all this together, do you also recommend the surgery?" I edged closer to the end of the stiff couch.

When the idea of surgery was initially proposed in Dr. Rodgers' office a little less than a year before, I was afraid of a procedure that would remove up to twenty percent of my brain. As the time passed, however, I understood that epilepsy surgery might be my best option if it offered the possibility of freedom from seizures. So I listened with disappointment when Dr. Shan explained that he believed surgery was not the best choice for me.

"You've only tried one medication to treat your epilepsy, Kristin." Dr. Shan sensed my disappointment as I listened. "To meet the criteria of medically intractable epilepsy, you must have tried and failed at least three medications before we seriously consider other options."

I recalled how I felt when I started taking carbamazepine for the first time after my diagnosis in high school. I remembered the mental haziness and almost paralyzing lethargy that remained until my body eventually accepted the foreign chemical as a welcome friend that assisted in my daily fight against seizures. "I struggled to adjust when I first started taking carbamazepine," I explained. "I need to do that two more times with two different medications before I'm considered a candidate for surgery?"

"Surgery wouldn't be easy either," Dr. Shan said with a long sigh. "Remember, you'd be left with a permanent defect in your visual field. Post-surgical patients also sometimes report persistent headaches or changes in their mood. There's a small risk of infection or stroke. And there's no guarantee that temporal lobe surgery will lead to a cure for your seizures," he looked at me, resigned. "I'm still hopeful that we can find a medication that works for you."

I listened attentively and hid my frustration when he gave me instructions to increase my carbamazepine to a dose that he hoped would stop the seizures. I smiled unconvincingly when he laid out plans to switch to a different anti-seizure medication if the first strategy failed. Inside, I was empty. I was keenly disappointed to come so far and found so little. I felt a little bit like Dorothy when the wizard told to her to go away.

I turned my focus back to Dr. Shan, who talked about the disposable parts of my brain, the expected somnolence, dizziness, or headaches that I may experience with mounting medication doses, and the possibility that despite all interventions, I may never be free of seizures.

Mom and I packed our bags in silence when we got back to the hotel. I knew that my epilepsy was a tremendous burden to her as well and she wished for a magic wand as much as I did. When I was a child, Mom was an expert at applying Band-Aids to scraped knees and fixed almost any childhood ailment with a hug. Her powerlessness at this time in my life was devastating. I'd heard her say more than once: "If we only hadn't wrapped you in a warm blanket before we took you to the hospital during that first seizure, this never would have happened." In reality, my mother's attention and quick-wittedness were life-saving on that fateful day, but maternal guilt can override all reasoning.

When we drove back through the hills of northwestern Wisconsin, the idyllic scenery was no longer as vibrant as before. The rolling landscape was washed with a gray dose of reality. The green pastures yellowed with fatigue. As we logged mile after mile, I turned my mind forward to focus on what was ahead instead of dwelling on the uncertainty of my condition. Not for the first time, I pulled myself into a public "Everything's okay" mode. The familiar deceptions I employed to re-create the outward appearance of normalcy and strength were so practiced that even my mother relaxed. I threw myself back into my normal routines so convincingly and surely that only I trembled with fear of what was to come.

* * *

E

Just as the medical community's knowledge about epilepsy has changed drastically over time, the available treatments for patients with epilepsy have diversified greatly over the centuries.

In the time before Hippocrates, when epilepsy was thought of as a sacred disease and seizures were a divine punishment for sinners, patients would offer sacrifices and take part in religious ceremonies in attempt to be cured. Later followers of Hippocrates prescribed a series of herbs, lifestyle modifications, and physiotherapy for treatment of seizures.[10]

In the 19th century, as neurology emerged as a new discipline distinct from psychiatry, the concept of epilepsy as a brain disorder became more widely accepted. Bromide, the world's first effective anti-epileptic medication, was introduced in 1857. Sir Charles Locock, Queen Victoria of England's obstetrician, announced at a meeting in 1857 that he had used potassium bromide to treat women with what he called hysterical epilepsy. Most of the seizures experienced by women with hysterical epilepsy occurred around the time of their menstrual cycle. Locock also took note of a German study, which demonstrated that a small amount of potassium bromide taken three times a day could cause reversible impotence.

When the same small dose of potassium bromide was given to women with hysterical epilepsy, Locock found that the frequency of their seizures decreased significantly.[11] After he noted these findings, bromide was increasingly used to treat cases of both menstrual and non-menstrual epilepsy during the second half of the 19th century. But as bromide's use increased, it was found to be ineffective in approximately 50% percent of patients with epilepsy, and associated with toxic side-effects such as irritability, emotional instability, impaired memory, headache, slurred speech, and an acne-like rash on the face and hands.[12]

13

TWO WEEKS AFTER Mom and I returned from our trip to Mayo Clinic, I started my second year of medical school. Surprisingly, the slightly increased dose of carbamazepine quelled my monthly cluster of seizures with only a few additional side effects. The second year of medical school offered a decreased workload and a predictable class schedule compared to first year. In class, I learned about the physiology of the human body one organ system at a time. Outside of the confines of medical school, my relationship with Andrew grew.

Andrew proposed early in the summer after my second year. In the early evening on that memorable day, we wandered slowly through the neighborhood grocery store and collected staples for a light picnic. We fanned our faces along with other shoppers to ward off the oppressive heat. Andrew accumulated a basketful of fruits and vegetables in atypical silence. I was used to him narrating every aspect of the day so it was unusual for him to be so quiet. For a fleeting moment, I wondered if something was amiss.

After paying for our groceries, we loaded them into the muted-green sedan that Andrew nicknamed "Kermit." Soon we were traveling on the undulating country roads near the Wisconsin River valley forty miles west of Madison. Andrew's familiar banter resumed. We commiserated about the pressures of graduate school while we drove—Andrew's business school studies and responsibilities easily paralleled the stress of medical school. A comfortable contentment spread over me like a warm blanket as we talked. I could rest in this place with him forever.

We pulled onto the gravel road leading to Bethel Horizons just as the sun began its descent to the fuchsia horizon. Bethel Horizons is a church retreat and nature center where Andrew spent weeks every summer growing up. It's unique for its miles of untouched land that encompasses pristine cliffs, valleys, natural ponds, and dramatic hills splashed with color by the native trees and wildflowers. We gathered our picnic supplies and hiked a circuitous trail through the prairie.

The summer sun had bleached the tall grass that carpeted the prairie. The friction from the brush, wilting wildflowers, and tall grasses hugging the small path scratched raw ruts in my legs. I neared exasperation when Andrew pointed out a small puddle of water made by a bubbling freshwater spring. Amidst the dryness of the heat-baked prairie, nature lured a bubbling fountain from the ground. I viewed it as a sign of new life.

The surrounding vegetation and topography changed quickly when we climbed the path to the cliff at the center of the park. Andrew and I said little and enjoyed the comfortable peace of companionship. I gazed over the steep precipice onto miles of uninterrupted fields and valleys below when we finally reached the top of the cliff. The view was testament to my insignificance in the vast, ever-changing universe.

Andrew interrupted my daydream, got down on one knee, and spoke quietly when he gently grasped my hand. We'd dated for years and had a multitude of conversations about what the future would bring. Finally I understood his recent silence, introspection, and kneeling posture. I admired the spark in his green eyes and anticipated the very question that emerged from his lips. "Kristin, will you marry me?"

The answer seemed obvious. "Yes!"

We embraced and wiped away tears of joy. When our love-struck gazes turned toward the valley, three majestic deer slowly stepped out of the forest and traversed the clearing beneath us. As soon as the deer moved back into the brush, a resplendent bald eagle swooped from one high treetop to another. We watched nature's dance in the clearing and felt that we were safe with each other, no matter what the future might bring.

*   *   *

During the third year of medical school, we finally had the opportunity to interact with real, live patients fighting real, live illnesses. I proudly dressed for work every morning in my white lab coat but felt perpetually inundated by the continuous flow of information about a smattering of medical specialties that never slowed or stopped.

During the first part of my third year, I spent two months each on rotations with internal medicine, family medicine, and surgery. My tasks during the day included participation with the team that took care of hospitalized patients, attendance of lectures on specialty-specific topics, and learning how to diagnose and manage a wide variety of illnesses. I found that while the opportunity to potentially "fix" a patient's problem in the operating room was fascinating, I had no desire to spend my days leaning over an anesthetized patient. Although the medically complex patients on the internal medicine service were an exciting challenge, the sickly adults didn't stir passion in me.

I was immediately inspired by the chance to make a positive change in a patient's wellbeing, however, when it came time to participate in the care of children. The added mystery of the developing human body and challenges offered by each child's varying ability to communicate had me hooked. Early in my third year, I decided I would be a pediatrician.

On an unexpectedly warm spring day near the end of my third year, I stepped out of the weathered door of my apartment with enthusiasm. The air blew fresh with energy and promise, a magician pulling off a delicious trick following the long darkness of winter. I eagerly anticipated my new rotation when I entered the familiar rotating doors of the University of Wisconsin Hospital.

The pediatric neurology service met on the fourth floor of the hospital. The pediatric ward was decorated with cheerful window paint and construction paper that soothed the sad, fearful faces of most of the young patients. Each morning, a team of white-coat clad physicians and medical students walked briskly down the hall behind an attending physician. The "attending"—or the physician ultimately responsible for the decisions that guided patient care—led the group with the harsh tap of his dress shoes and his chin pointed toward the ceiling decorated with construction paper birds and butterflies. A team of medical students and residents spread out behind him like a flock of migrating birds in formation. The long white coats of the first year residents were weighed down with medical tools, notes, and a plethora of crumpled papers filled with information about their patients. Pagers hung precariously from the cinched waists of their wrinkled scrubs and dark circles framed their eyes, melding with the haggard lines and creases imprinted by fatigue. Although I was anxious to join the ranks of the residents, who'd only recently graduated from medical school, I didn't dare look that far ahead.

We medical students followed timidly behind the residents with our clipboards raised protectively like shields. We stepped quickly in formation with our eyes downcast. Some of us had noses buried in one of several pocket books of quick reference for neurological diseases. I glided along with the group, thrilled to be part of the motley crew but terrified of making the wrong impression.

I was eager to learn about pediatric neurology from the other side. Some of the children on the ward were recovering from seizures like I experienced as a child. I hoped to learn more about the physiology of seizures and epilepsy. I dreamt that I might find a hidden treatment for my seizures sequestered somewhere in the construction paper-lined hallways.

While we migrated down the long corridor, I listened as the resident briefed the group on the next patient. "This is a six-year-old female with Lennox-Gastaut Syndrome and recurrent seizures that have been refractory to all medications so far. As you know, Lennox-Gastaut Syndrome is a severe form of epilepsy associated with multiple different seizure types, developmental delay, and behavioral disturbances. She is here for initiation of the ketogenic diet."

The resident, Sameer, spoke with confidence as he updated the group on his patient's status. I wondered if a small portion of success in medicine was obtained by cultivating the ability to act confident even when filled with self-doubt.

Sameer stopped outside the patient's room and turned to face us. He carefully checked the small note card in his white coat pocket. "We're working with the G.I. team to make sure that she's maintaining adequate nutrition while starting this special diet. The patient's current medications are lamictal, keppra, and diazepam as needed."

One by one, our group entered the patient's room to check on her status and meet with her parents. We found a small girl lying twisted on the large hospital bed, her expression muted by the confusion that accumulates with severe, recurrent seizures. Laura turned up her lips in a brief, fleeting smile in response to our appearance before she returned to her world of bewilderment. Her hands were flexed tightly into her armpits and her thin legs resembled sinew-covered bird legs instead of the fleshy extremities of a six-year-old child. Laura watched expectantly as her father crossed the room to talk with us.

I inwardly wept at how Laura's unrelenting seizures had transformed an innocent little girl with golden curls into a fragile porcelain doll. My seizures frustrated me and fed a brewing uneasiness. Laura's seizures, however, were transformative and devastating. I had a new appreciation for the wrath that epilepsy can leave in its wake. I took notes diligently and made a mental note to study more about Lennox-Gastaut Syndrome and the ketogenic diet.

Later I learned that the ketogenic diet is a very specific diet used for treatment of severe, difficult-to-control epilepsy that mimics starvation and forces the body to burn fats instead of carbohydrates. When there are little to no carbohydrates in the diet, the liver converts fats to fatty acids and ketones. An elevated level of ketones, or the energy source that the body produces in states of starvation or stress, is associated with reduction of seizures in some children.

As I left the room with the rest of the neurology team, I thought that in a significant way, Laura and I were kin. It seemed that we would resort to almost anything, whether dramatic diets, potent medications, or surgery, to make our seizures disappear forever.

*   *   *

Halfway into my pediatric neurology rotation, I met a patient who made me feel like I was staring into the rearview mirror. Melanie Dodge was a perfect three-year-old girl. She loved to spend summer days outside collecting colorful pebbles and playing ballerina while clad in pink skirts and tutus. Melanie was the first child in her family, but her mother's belly was blossoming with the brother they expected the following month. Melanie enjoyed an illness-free first three years of life until the day before I met her.

The previous morning, Melanie hosted a pretend tea party with her friends and dolls when her posture transformed from relaxed and happy to rigid and fixed. She froze with an unrecognizable look on her face that registered somewhere between panic and confusion.

"Melanie?" The girls' mothers had been chatting nearby. When there was no response, her mother jumped up, alarmed. "Melanie!"

The child answered her mother's call with an eerie noise that reverberated around the room. She fell to the floor wildly twitching and stiffening with the characteristic rhythmic muscle contractions that are typical of a grand mal seizure.

Melanie's mother called 9-1-1 for help but the details of the events after that were all a blur. She remembered that the convulsions were relentless and continued forever. Melanie's chart said that the total duration of her first seizure was just under an hour.

I met Melanie and Mrs. Dodge for the first time when Melanie was sedated in the pediatric intensive care unit. The lines and tubes that coiled from her small body created a fishnet of medical security.

Just as when I was a toddler, massive amounts of sedatives were administered the night before to quell the all-consuming electrical storm. While the ventilator rhythmically puffed air into Melanie's lungs, her mother sat steadfastly by her bedside, unknowingly breathing in rhythm with the steely vent.

The scene was hauntingly familiar. Twenty-two years before, it was my body lying unmoving in a similar hospital bed. My mother remained perpetually by my side until I returned to the carefree toddler she knew. A chill ran up my spine as I understood some of the distress and pain that Melanie's mother, and mine, felt from their vantage point next to a fallen child.

The pediatric neurology team discussed Melanie in the same business-like fashion that we used when conversing about all of the other neurology patients on the ward. I was the student assigned to Melanie's team, so it was my job to introduce the patient and review the events that happened overnight. When it came time to present to the team, I struggled to speak even though I was prepared after forty minutes of studying Melanie's chart. I was distracted by the persistent and nagging hope that things would be different for Melanie than they were for me.

Though eventually I presented my patient in a somewhat intelligent and organized manner, my mind wandered. My first seizure occurred over twenty years ago, but the medical management of prolonged seizures—or status epilepticus—was disturbingly unchanged. I was outwardly successful and on my way to achieving my life goals, but I still lived with fear of seizures every day. Considering Melanie and my shared history, I wasn't sure if my history could serve as a positive example or an omen.

I never shared my story with Melanie and her family. I didn't want to alarm them with the truth of what life might be like for their tiny daughter. But, I was also more comfortable in my medical student role. It was easier to walk down the hall with the same confidence as my classmates if no one else knew that I, too, could dip into a state of "impaired consciousness" at any minute. My white coat and clipboard rendered me relatively invincible from the lapping unpredictability of chronic illness. Only time would tell when my pride would come crashing down.

* * *

E

Seizures with fever, or febrile seizures, are very common in young children and almost always benign. They are most commonly seen in children between the ages of six months and five years and are thought to occur in otherwise healthy children when the rapid rise in temperature interrupts the electrical activity of the brain. Although two to four percent of children under the age of five will have a febrile seizure, the risk of recurrence is highest in infants under the age of one year.[13]

Febrile seizures are classified as "simple" or "complex" based on the nature of the seizure. Complex febrile seizures—like the ones Melanie and I had—may last more than 15 minutes, occur more than once in 24 hours, or involve only one side of the body. In contrast, simple febrile seizures are shorter, involve full body movements and complete loss of consciousness, and do not recur within a short time frame.

Children with a history of simple febrile seizures have only a slightly increased risk of developing epilepsy compared to the general population.[14] Although there appears to be an association between prolonged febrile seizures and hippocampal sclerosis, it isn't completely known whether the hippocampal changes are due to prolonged seizures or causative of them.[15] The possible link between prolonged febrile seizures and temporal lobe epilepsy is an active area of epilepsy research.

14
2000

ANDREW AND I MARRIED in June during a whirlwind three weeks between the third and fourth year of medical school. In the days prior to our wedding, my parents' house filled with my brothers and their wives, grandparents, aunts, uncles, and friends from all over the world. I basked in the glow of the familiar nest of love that I'd left behind to navigate the challenges of medical school.

Our wedding day arrived with a warmth and grey mist of humidity that hovered over the manicured lawns of our neighborhood as far as the eye could see. The heavy clouds hung low and threatened to rain through our outdoor pictures, during the jubilant ride to church, and when I walked gingerly in my pristine ivory dress across the gravel parking lot to the open church doors. Though my heart fluttered with a combination of nervousness and excitement, I knew the sanctuary was filled with the people who mattered most to us.

My childhood piano teacher, Mrs. Busse, sat at the organ awaiting our arrival. Andrew's host dad from Japan played a melodious version of Clair de Lune on the grand piano. Former classmates from the Lutheran Campus Center made up a choir that sang throughout the service. The pastor from Bethel Horizons stood in front to officiate.

My childhood friends Wendy and Laura joined my college room-mates Sapna and Colene in matching lavender bridesmaid dresses.

When it was finally time to march down the aisle, I could hardly contain my excitement and joy. My smile was wide enough to make my lips shake and my cheeks ache. I progressed with such cer-tainty that the photographer tapped me on the shoulder and gently reminded me to slow down.

When Andrew and I exchanged our vows, I heard the firm cadence of raindrops on the roof. I stole a glimpse out a near window and watched a child sprint across the parking lot while trying to avoid the downpour. By the time the service was over and it was time to go outside, the only remnants of the rain were the shiny, wet blacktop and the double rainbow forming above.

Andrew and I watched the colors form in the sky. The beauty of the rainbows felt like an otherworldly blessing, like the stately deer that marched across the prairie when he proposed. Later at our reception, Andrew's host mom from Tokyo reminded us that in Japan, rain on a wedding day is considered good luck. When we mingled with the guests and ate appetizers, the couple who was celebrating their fiftieth anniversary in the party room below stepped onto the outside balcony and shouted their blessings and best wishes for the years ahead. Little did we know we would need all the good wishes and luck we could find.

*   *   *

The American Grizzly bear spends hours each fall consuming large amounts of food to prepare for a long winter rest. As the days become shorter and colder, the bears search for a den where they can sleep for most of the winter months. They curl into tight balls for warmth while their heart rates slow and their body temperatures drop several degrees. The bears aren't true hibernators because they occasionally wake and wander out of their dens during the winter, but they do very little before the spring brings warm breezes and sunlight back to the horizon.

Like the Grizzly, my seizures hibernated through the wonderful early years of my marriage to Andrew, fourth year and subsequent graduation from medical school, and through the beginning of my pediatric residency. I don't exactly remember when epilepsy returned, but soon enough I began waking with unexplained bite marks on the side of my tongue, the characteristic sign of a nocturnal seizure. Inspecting my tongue became part of my morning ritual. Each morning I showered, brushed my teeth, combed my hair, and checked my tongue. It wasn't long before I found that the marks appeared with increasing frequency. Soon, the rekindled complex partial seizures spilled into the daytime hours as well. Sleepless nights were common and 100-hour workweeks were the norm in the first year of my pediatric residency. The exhaustion and stress of residency woke my hibernating bear from its slumber.

Since my seizures came in clusters, the presence or absence of bite marks came to predict whether I was going to have a good or bad day. On a "bad" day, I worried that every unusual feeling, fleeting headache, or momentary bit of indigestion signaled a looming seizure. Despite all of my watchfulness, the seizures usually caught me when I least expected them. They came while I was dressing in the morning, when I walked down the long sterile ward at the hospital, or while I documented a patient's chart at the end of the day.

When I visited Dr. Rodgers again in the middle of my first year of pediatric residency, he suggested that it was time to try a different seizure medication. The increased dose of carbamazepine recommended by Dr. Shan at Mayo had been helpful for years, but it was no longer effective even at the highest possible dose. We couldn't tell if this was secondary to the stress and erratic lifestyle of my residency, or if I'd developed a higher propensity toward seizures. A newer medication on the market, called lamotrigine, showed some success in treatment of complex partial seizures. I was eager to give it a try.

The process of switching from one anti-epileptic medication to another was anything but simple. Dr. Rodgers introduced me to Mitch Caros, a pharmacist who specialized in the treatment of neurologic disorders. Mitch detailed the step-by-step approach I'd follow to wean off carbamazepine and switch to lamotrigine.

With triangular glasses hanging at the tip of his nose, Mr. Caros looked over my chart and fired questions at me as if I were at a job interview. "I see you've used carbamazepine with the addition of diamox around your menses. Have you tried any other anti-epileptic medications?"

"No, that's it," I replied.

Mr. Caros rubbed his bearded face and studied me. "Did you have any trouble tolerating carbamazepine?"

"I was exhausted when I first started it." I worried that I couldn't maintain my challenging residency schedule if I had the same reaction to a new medication. "After awhile it was okay."

Mr. Caros sat up straight in his chair and began, "Lamotrigine, or lamictal, has some chemical differences from carbamazepine but the same desired effect. It's a good choice for treatment of temporal lobe seizures.

"There's a very small chance that you may develop a rash when you start taking lamotrigine. The rash is an allergic reaction that may start as small red dots but in rare cases may lead to blistering of your skin, mouth, and even eyes. This blistering type of rash may be life-threatening. If you notice any skin changes when you start taking lamotrigine, please contact us immediately."

Mr. Caros went on to explain the myriad of other possible side effects that could occur with ingestion of lamotrigine. There were way too many potential side effects to really remember. I resigned to wait and see what the new medication had in store for me.

Finally, Mr. Caros gave me a printed list of the points we discussed and the appointment was over. I drove home with my head tilted back on the headrest and the radio tuned to classical music to quiet my mind. Although glad to take a step to reduce my seizures, I felt troubled by the reminder that I may never find the magic solution. Other than the handful of medications that bookended my days, I could go weeks at a time forgetting about epilepsy. When I walked through the hospital as a resident physician with growing authority, it was hard to remember that I also belonged to the same corridors as a patient. The reminder that I, too, was just a seizure away from becoming a defenseless patient unearthed the very roots of my confidence.

At home that night, I pulled my favorite pillow next to the gas fireplace and sat where I could appreciate the intensity of the heat. I held one of my medical textbooks and struggled to concentrate while my mind danced like the flames around the fear of the unknown. After a while, I called my mom. We talked about my residency rotations, the new condo Andrew and I had recently acquired, and the reality of starting over with a new anti-epileptic medication.

Mom's empathy wrapped around me like a virtual hug. I fell asleep that night feeling safe in the sheath of love that protected me. Andrew cradled me in the shelter of his warm arms each evening while my parents and family spun webs of sanctuary from their homes nearby. My resident colleagues and comrades buoyed me with their love and support. I was acutely aware of what a tremendous blessing it was to have all of these cheerleaders nearby. If I remained focused, with my doctor and patient identities stabilized and delicately aligned, it was impossible to sink.

*   *   *

E

In the early part of the 20ᵗʰ century, phenobarbital, an anti-epileptic drug that's still used today, was introduced. The ability to measure the serum levels of anti-epileptic drugs was also explored during this period. It became clear that a relationship existed between blood levels and effectiveness and also toxicity of each medication. Physicians of the early 20ᵗʰ century also began to focus on how epilepsy could be affected by other aspects of a patient's life. Careful attendance to these details was thought to contribute to treatment of seizures. In the mid-1930s, neurologist Samuel Alexander Kinnier Wilson wrote:

> "Irregularities of faults in the patient's mode of life must be put right. He should be allowed his share of games and recreations even at some little risk, unless this is known to be deleterious. The salutary and bracing effect of being considered 'normal' must be balanced against the danger (should it be present) of over-exertion."

From the 1930s until today, multiple new medications have been introduced for treatment of seizures. As researchers have described the electromagnetic processes that lead to normal electric messages in the brain, medications have been developed to target specific steps in the cascade where conduction can go awry and lead to a seizure. Though medications developed more recently are increasingly potent and specific, all are associated with significant side effects. Commonly found are fatigue, nausea, cognitive side effects, or problems with balance. Though there are now 26 anti-epileptic drugs, one third of epilepsy patients continue to have seizures despite medications.

15

THE NEXT MORNING, I swallowed one small pink tablet along with my usual three pale pink capsules, pushed back my sense of doubt, and pasted on my best smile. I focused my gaze at the picturesque Wisconsin Capitol building, a perfect white dome in the middle of a green island, while Andrew drove me to the work. Soon the brown cluster of hexagonal pods known as the University of Wisconsin hospital came into my view, the first commute safely behind me. At least for the first few hours, my new medication hadn't caused any adverse effects. I began just another regular day.

Over the next several weeks, I slowly increased the dose of one medication while decreasing the other. I was more tired than usual, but truly no more than my normal post-call state. Residency already taught me to function through a constant low-level exhaustion. I considered it a victory when I finally reached the target dose of lamotrigine without an outward sign of the fluctuating medication levels.

Soon enough, however, my seizures returned. At first, they were intermittent and sporadic. Before long, I expected uninvited interruptions to my day or sleep every one to two weeks. I expressed concern during my next appointment with Dr. Rodgers. "What now?" I asked as I studied the walls lined with enlarged pictures of anti-epileptic medications.

Dr. Rodgers perused the pack of my medical records. He contemplated my options for a long time and finally recommended that I try treatment with oxcarbamazapine, or Carbatrol, next.

The pharmacist Mitch Caros appeared within minutes to guide me through the switch from lamotrigine to oxcarbamazepine. Again he recited a list of daunting potential side effects, including dizziness, drowsiness, fatigue, nausea, insomnia, acne, or constipation. I wore a noncommittal gaze while my mind ventured into the world of unknowns and possibilities. What if this medication didn't work either? What if it did? What would it take to send my seizures back into hibernation?

The following morning, I swallowed the first dose of my newest medication with a belly full of hope. I arrived at work early to review the charts and overnight events on a large group of hematology/oncology patients before the attending doctors came in. As the first year resident, it was my job to review the medications, vital signs, laboratory values, and progress made in the previous 24 hours so the medical team could make decisions and guide care for the new day. I sat in a small conference room the size of a compact minivan and realized that I was jotting notes not with one pencil, but two. Instead of focusing on one computer monitor in front of me, I saw two. Alarmed, I spun around to look outside the conference room door where the mother of one of my patients—and her phantom counterpart—stood in the doorway with a concerned look on her face. She'd spent the night in the hospital room with her child, so she was still dressed in flannel pajama pants and brown footie slippers. Her hands were huddled around her large mug of coffee as if it were a campfire.

"How are you today, Dr. Seaborg? You look tired."

"I am," I responded. How could I explain that I was starting a new medication, seeing double, and yet participating in the care of her child?

"I was just wondering if you had the results of Cody's lab tests yet?"

I typed my password and username into the computer with considerable effort and found Cody's most recent lab results. With one eye closed, my vision wasn't as bad. I reviewed the daily blood counts with Cody's mother and breathed a sigh of relief when I watched the cotton tassels on her slippers pad back down the hall.

The morning crept on, and I slowly collected data from the computer in my one-eyed ogre stance while the tiny room filled with a menagerie of medical students, residents, and attending physicians.

With my pre-rounding work done, I sat on a cushioned bench in the crowded conference room and waited for rounds to begin. Abruptly, a familiar sensation engulfed me. First I swallowed repetitively, then I flushed warm with more swallowing. Next I smacked my lips and my whole face felt as if it were on fire. Although I was acutely aware that something was amiss, the subtle motions of my smacking lips and recurrent swallowing went unnoticed by the other members of the busy medical team. The unpleasant feelings of my complex partial seizure crescendoed and then decrescendoed until finally I wished I could curl up and fall asleep.

The seizure abated after a minute or more. As I regained full awareness, I looked up and saw the tail of the white coat of Dr. Isaac, the pediatric neurosurgeon, flutter into the room as if he were an angel.

Through my double vision and post-seizure cloudy thinking, my only coherent thought was: I needed to have epilepsy surgery to find a cure. I cared for dozens of patients collaboratively with Dr. Isaac and admired his sense of commitment, sincerity, and expertise.

So I looked up at the two Dr. Isaacs who stood next to me and asked, "Do you do temporal lobectomies?"

Confusion painted his face. "Yes. Why?"

"I think I need one."

The floodgates opened and I tripped over my words as I tried to explain what I'd been through in the past six months, much less the past twenty-five years, I brushed aside my secrecy and pride when I pleaded for help while sitting amongst ten people who knew nothing about my health history.

"My neurologist says that I have temporal lobe epilepsy and a focal lesion that can be removed surgically, but I've been trying medications first. I've switched medicines now three times in three months. Today I'm seeing double and I feel terrible. Just now I had another complex partial seizure. Nothing is working and I think I just need to go ahead and get this over with.

"Can you help me?"

* * *

E

One in 26 people will develop epilepsy at some point during their lifetime. In fact, epilepsy affects over three million Americans of all ages, which makes it more common than cerebral palsy, multiple sclerosis, muscular dystrophy, and Parkinson's Disease *combined*. In America, epilepsy is as common as breast cancer, and claims just as many lives. The mortality rate amongst patients with epilepsy is two-to-three times higher than the general population. The risk of sudden death amongst those with epilepsy is 24 times greater.[16]

Epilepsy costs the United States $15.5 billion each year. In reality, the indirect costs associated with uncontrolled seizures are seven times higher than those of the average of *all* chronic diseases.[17] Despite these astounding statistics, research in epilepsy has been historically underfunded. The National Institutes of Health (NIH) spends $30 billion annually on medical research but only 0.5% of NIH funds are allocated for research in epilepsy.

Part II: The Patient

16
2002

THUNDERSTORMS START from a rapid, upward movement of warm, moist air. As the air moves upwards, it cools, condenses, and forms towering cumulonimbus clouds. The action of rising and descending air within a thunderstorm separates positive and negative discharges. Lightning results from the buildup and discharge of electrical energy between positively charged areas. The effects of thunderstorms, such as high winds, hail, heavy precipitation and tornadoes, can be extremely dangerous.

When my seizures spun beyond control, I felt as volatile as the swirling electric air that mounts within a thunderstorm. I started on my quest to seek a stable atmosphere of calm to protect myself from the impending storm.

I trudged to my next visit with Dr. Rodgers resigned but resolute. I raised a white flag to epilepsy and surrendered my stoicism, stubbornness, and belief that I could do this all on my own. The encroaching walls of the corridor leading to the Neurology department left little room for air when I made my way down to the medical suite I knew too well.

Dr. Rodgers came through the exam room door stripped of his usual energy. "We really put you through the ringer," he admitted. I swallowed the lump in my throat and nodded assent. "How are you feeling?"

"Better," I offered. "Double vision isn't fun."

The morning that I started oxcarbamazepine and immediately experienced double vision and a complex partial seizure, several fellow residents escorted me to the quiet resident break room to rest. One of my colleagues rubbed my back while I held my head in my hands and another found Dr. Rodger's office number. Dr. Rodgers' nurse, Karen, instructed me to discontinue the offensive oxcarbamazepine and gradually increase lamotrigine back to an effective dose. Andrew picked me up from work and escorted me home where I fell quickly into a deep, disturbed sleep.

"I'm glad you called that day. How are you tolerating the lamotrigine now?"

"Just fine."

"We should add another medication in addition to what you're taking now for better control of your seizures," Dr. Rodgers ventured.

Afraid to spin the medication roulette again, I interrupted. "I think it's time to talk about the surgery."

The night before, I'd had a frank conversation with both Andrew and my parents about how I felt each time I started a new medication and what surgery might offer. Those closest to my heart promised to support whatever decision I made. Andrew couldn't attend my midday appointment with Dr. Rodgers, but his affirmation and promise to stand by me "in sickness or in health" was comforting.

Dr. Rodgers wasn't surprised at all. I wondered if he'd long expected me to come to this inevitable conclusion. He grabbed his pen and began to list the things that needed to happen before the surgery could proceed. "We'll need to arrange for inpatient EEG monitoring," he said. "Our best monitoring unit is at the V.A. hospital, so I'll arrange for your admission there. Because we want to pinpoint the exact location of your seizures, you'll need to have intracranial electrodes placed prior to the video monitoring."

Dr. Rodgers paused and pointed to the side of his face just in front of his ear. "The insertion of the electrodes can be quite painful since they have to travel through the facial nerve to get to the space just underneath your temporal lobe. The facial nerve is a large nerve that provides sensation and movement to most of your face." He continued to point just above his jawline on the side of his face. "Unfortunately they have to keep you awake without pain medications during the procedure so the radiologist can ensure the electrodes get to the correct place."

I nodded, unfazed. The path that led to this point had been filled with obstacles and potholes. I didn't expect the next steps to be without challenges.

"We have a fairly recent MRI and PET scan, so I don't think that we need to repeat these.

"You'll also need to have a Wada test done. This is a procedure where we anesthetize one hemisphere of your brain at a time in attempt to locate where the foci for language and memory are."

This sounded alarming.

"And I'll need to present your case at the epilepsy conference to see if my colleagues agree that you are a candidate for epilepsy surgery."

I found my voice and asked, "How long do you think all of this will take?"

"It's October now," Dr. Rodgers studied a nearby calendar. "Usually the pre-op testing takes six months or longer. If everything goes as planned, you can anticipate surgery this spring.

"In the meantime, let's see if we can control your seizures by adding an additional medication. Levetiracetam, or Keppra, often works well in conjunction with other anti-epileptic drugs and with minimal side effects."

I was a fan of minimal side effects. My epilepsy was public knowledge amongst my resident colleagues now that I'd experienced double vision, numbing fatigue, and seizures in the workplace. I hoped to portray a semblance of life returning to normal.

I walked out of the neurology suite with appointment slips and phone numbers to call to begin pre-operative testing. I finally exhaled and allowed myself to breathe again when I reached the safety and shelter of the dank parking lot.

Medical school and residency taught me the importance of appearing worry-free without revealing my thoughts and feelings. The few times that I let my resolve crumble, such as the morning of my double vision, others viewed me as weak and vulnerable. Eighty percent of my job description as a pediatric resident was to remain strong and untouchable while those around me bled, cried, got sicker, and sometimes died.

In the small exam rooms of the neurology clinic, my "doctor" walls crumbled and I confronted not only my own fear, but also the vulnerability of the patients whom I cared for every day. In my defenselessness, I struggled to reconcile the two warring parts of me. I wanted to care for others, but I also wanted to be cared for. Underneath my outer shell, there was a struggling patient who searched for a gleaming light to guide my ship safely out of the tumultuous sea of seizures. My friends and family buoyed me up, but I still felt like I was floating alone against a current of chaos, poisonous chemicals ingested to quell the seizures, and an uncertain future. I strived to be a good doctor, but I could only become a better physician after I passed the test of being a humble patient.

Through the veil of exhaust in the parking garage, I studied the cars around me and concluded that the blessing hidden within my upcoming surgical experience was perspective. When I'd walked the same road as my patients, I'd be one step closer to becoming a compassionate physician.

*   *   *

When residents were assigned to be on call in the Pediatric Intensive Care Unit (PICU), we stayed overnight in a small, cramped call room in the hospital and spent many sleepless hours standing over the beds of the smallest, most fragile patients in the Children's Hospital. I was on call one night shortly before my scheduled inpatient stay for EEG monitoring.

Six-month-old Isabella was rolled into the PICU at the start of my shift. A grimace marred her porcelain face and tears lingered just beyond the ridges of her closed, almond-shaped eyes. No one was entirely sure what'd happened to Isabella. Her stepfather trailed close behind the moving gurney and recalled the events when she fell off the couch onto the carpeted floor hours before.

"She was lying next to me when, suddenly, it happened!" he exclaimed, looking away. "She rolled over and fell to the floor before I could catch her. As soon as she fell, she stopped crying. She's been like this ever since." Isabella's stepfather's face twisted with pain and he cast his guilty eyes to the floor to avoid our suspicious glares.

The child's arms and legs remained limp as we checked her radial, brachial, and femoral pulses and tried to rouse her from her deep sleep. An endotracheal tube sprouted from the crevasse between Isabella's crimson lips and a crescent of soft belly peeked from underneath the rim of her faded pink T-shirt. Intravenous lines were placed, her abdomen prodded, her clothes removed, but Isabella didn't respond.

Isabella's stepfather was ushered to a family waiting room while we continued to work to stabilize her and determine our next steps. My job as the junior resident was to perform a full admission physical exam. Her infant heart beat slowly but reliably and her lungs filled rhythmically with clear air as the ventilator breathed for her.

A shock of dark, wavy hair had tumbled down to mesh with the long, curled eyelashes that fringed her closed eyelids. I raised one lifeless lid to examine her pupillary reflexes and was frightened by an image that will forever remain in my memory.

The ophthalmoscope I used to examine Isabella's eyes is a tool that gives the examiner a clear view of the retina, where tiny vessels run like rivers to the optic nerve before it escapes through the back of the orbit on its journey to the brain. I was accustomed to seeing a handful of blood vessels similar to thin red snakes swimming toward the pale optic disc at the center of the view. But when I looked into Isabella's eyes, I found a threatening field of red splashed across the normally clear space. The image in Isabella's other eye was the very same—a stark crimson canvas that indicated the fragile retinal blood vessels were sheared and broken with tremendous force.

Isabella's retinal hemorrhages were the hallmark sign that she'd been shaken so forcefully that her brain was now irreparably damaged. I was horrified that a beautiful, perfect infant marched toward the irreversible diagnosis of brain death. Suddenly her stepfather's odd behavior and inability to meet our eyes made sense. The baby's small neurons couldn't withstand the power of an enraged adult shaking her body like a rag doll. I took a deep breath and fought back welling tears while I gently closed Isabella's eyes and said a silent prayer.

Isabella didn't die that night. The ventilator and IV fluids kept her body alive until an EEG confirmed the diagnosis of brain death. Isabella's stepfather admitted that he shook her out of frustration when she was crying, and he was subsequently taken into custody. Several days later, her mother agreed to withdraw life support once it was clear that Isabella would never survive her injury. In a last beautiful gesture, her organs were donated to sustain the lives of several other much more fortunate children.

But during that awful night in the PICU, I was far from welcoming the comfort of the morning sun. As soon as I walked out of Isabella's room in anger and sorrow, I was called down the hall to check on Makayla.

Makayla was a four-year-old with symmetric braids of thick black hair and glistening dimples that marked the middle of her cavernous cheeks. She was diagnosed with a pediatric tumor of the eye called retinoblastoma two years previously, shortly after her father passed away from the same disease. Makayla's initial round of surgery and chemotherapy was successful, even though one of her bright, mahogany eyes was removed to rid her body of the tumor. Several months before her admission to the PICU, Makayla began complaining of pain in her hip and neck. A CT scan confirmed metastasis of her original tumor to several areas throughout her body.

When I entered Makayla's hospital room, she was curled tightly in her mother's lap. Her mother shielded her protectively with her long arms and strong shoulders. Though she cradled her baby in a loving embrace, a mother's love wasn't enough to reverse the slow decline in Makayla's heart rate and shallow breathing. Makayla's cancer had advanced inexorably enough that she was losing her grasp on life. A nurse was present to administer medications to ease her passage into another world. It would be my job to pronounce her dead.

Makayla's mother wept quietly as she held her baby and monitored the florescent green line that recorded her heart rate on a monitor nearby. I stood discretely in the corner and tried to blend in with the wallpaper, feeling like I was eavesdropping on an intensely personal moment. A hospice nurse held Makayla's mother's hand. Her gentle sobs became louder each time the child's fragile breathing slowed. Makayla's bright fingernails, polished a fire engine red, seemed out of place in the somber room.

We stood that way for what seemed like forever. At last, Makayla took a final sigh to announce that she'd fought long enough. The bouncing green line flattened, and the child's mother wailed and cradled her daughter close to her cheek and cried, "My baby my baby my baby." I made a note in Makayla's chart. Time of death: 12:03 A.M. Death was stronger than a pristine child with bright red fingernails and an insatiable cancer.

The familiar vibration of the pager on my belt abruptly pulled me from my thoughts. The story ended in Makayla's room, but down the hall, the Med Flight team wheeled in another patient in need of acute care. I jogged down the curved hallway and found the attending physician talking quickly to the assembled group at the same time he used an inflatable bag and mask to breathe for an unconscious patient.

"Sixteen-year-old female who ran into a tree while skiing in a race approximately two hours ago. The victim was wearing a helmet but the helmet was crushed during headfirst impact with the tree. The patient was found unconscious and unresponsive on the hill and no longer breathing independently. She was intubated immediately and flown here."

I studied the patient's condition while I listened.

"In-flight management included ventilation and fluid resuscitation. So far, we haven't been able to get any purposeful responses with stimulation. She has an open head wound with visible extruding white matter. Brain swelling and cerebellar herniation are a significant concern."

As soon as the gurney stopped, a swarm of doctors and nurses flocked to the patient. "Let's move her over." Dr. Brady, the attending PICU physician, gestured to the larger bed in the hospital room.

"On my count. 1-2-3!"

We slid the patient as gingerly as possible to the bed that would become her home for the next three weeks. I inspected the devastated teenager lying before me as the energy and chaos in the room calmed.

Sarah was sixteen but she didn't look a day over twelve, even when shroud with a cluster of medical devices, splints, and dried blood. A turban of bloody gauze clung to her head, and her neck and body were strapped to a rigid board to ensure stability of her spine. Sarah's eyes were small slits of eyelashes hidden in a sea of swelling and bruises that'd previously been her youthful face. There were several untouched locks of caramel-colored hair that escaped and flowed down to her shoulders just outside the rigid confines of the cervical collar and head dressing. Looped purple pen strokes marked an unknown phone number on her hand, a remnant of the carefree teenage existence that was crushed to pieces along with her skull against that tree.

We hooked Sarah to the monitors and ventilator in the ICU and inspected her wounds while we waited for the neurosurgery team. She would need emergency surgery to stabilize the swelling in her brain and decompress her skull fracture. We watched her vital signs with trepidation.

Moments later, I tore my eyes away from the monitors around Sarah's bed and turned to see a cluster of neurosurgeons jogging down the narrow path to the ICU. Their white coats floated behind them as if they were galloping on clouds as they pushed forward to the girl's room. My shoulders relaxed and my breathing eased when the neurosurgery team wheeled Sarah down the hall to the operating room. Isabella and Makayla wouldn't live to see adulthood, but Sarah's future remained a possibility. For this, at least, I was hopeful.

In one night, I met the Unimaginable, Unavoidable, and the Unexpected. Three beautiful girls' lives altered or ceased while most of Madison slept. Weeping, I walked the lakeshore path in the morning sun as I left the hospital. I cried in frustration at how helpless I could be even when cast in the "helper" role. I was also ashamed of my obsession with my own illness. Seizures were frustrating and unpredictable, but I still woke each morning to welcome the promise of a new day. Anticipation and expectation were still mine to enjoy. Isabella, Makayla, and Sarah now embodied only golden memories or fiery regrets of moments gone tragically awry. I dried my tears and lifted my chin to the sun as I filled my lungs with the cool, early spring air. It was a new day, and I was acutely grateful to be part of the world.

17
2003

THE WILLIAM S. MIDDLETON Veteran's Hospital in Madison is nationally recognized for its high quality of care. I walked into the vast hospital lobby on the day of my admission for prolonged video EEG monitoring, passing several small clusters of veterans and visitors huddled over plates of doughnuts and pots of coffee. Andrew and I followed the gleaming white path to the Admissions desk and waited patiently for the clerk to look up from his computer. After what seemed like an unconscionably long time, the clerk looked up and grunted, "Can I help you?"

The man was looking directly at Andrew with expectation. Andrew quickly caught the mistake. "My wife is the patient," he said, pointing to me.

The man at the computer shook off a surprised look and quickly redirected his dull brown eyes toward me. "Can I help you?" he asked again.

"I'm here to check in," I said. "I'm scheduled for inpatient EEG monitoring."

The clerk paused for a moment and thought out loud. "You don't look like the typical patient around here."

I let the comment drop, answering instead with a smile and nod. It would be an interesting few days.

The man gave Andrew and me directions to my room in such an eloquent manner that it seemed like we'd checked into a hotel. We rode the elevator up with an amputee in a wheelchair, a man with a tracheotomy and accompanying oxygen tank, and a cart of bland food packaged for lunch on the sixth floor.

We stepped off into the general neurology unit when the elevator finally opened at the eighth floor. We walked down the checked linoleum corridor already scrubbed and sterilized to a uniform, grey color. I turned into room 8159 and studied the small, rectangular space that would become my home for the next week. First, I noticed the surprising, majestic view of the frozen Lake Mendota from the picture window across the room. The barren landscape below was dotted with colorful shacks that belonged to ice fishers brave enough to spend a day outside in the below-zero cold.

My gaze traveled along the walls of the hospital room. The hair on my neck rose when I spotted a camera trained on the bed along with the wires and materials needed to record an EEG. I took a deep breath and wondered again what lay ahead.

Only seconds after Andrew set my suitcase down on the tired linoleum floor, a large man clad in bright turquoise scrubs blew into the room. "Mr. Seaborg," he spoke in a loud, booming voice. "I see you're here for an inpatient EEG."

Andrew pointed my way again. "She's the patient."

The turquoise-shroud nurse didn't hide his surprise. "Well, um, Mrs. Seaborg, I'm here to place your IV."

Nurse Blue headed purposefully toward the hospital bed in the center of the room where I was sitting. He grabbed my arm and searched for favorable veins. After a few minutes of searching, he was satisfied with a vein that travelled like a thick blue yarn on top of my left hand. He paused to gather his materials and an angiocath, clear tape, tourniquet, and adhesive tape inexplicably materialized from his deep blue pocket. He arranged everything neatly in a line and finally turned toward me to initiate some by-the-book small talk.

Up close, I noticed beads of sweat forming on his broad forehead and small flecks of spittle that flew far from his mouth with each consonant. "Are you from the Madison area?" The spit flew from his mouth to my forearm held down in position for the IV.

"I've been living here for the past ten years," I responded. "But I grew up in a suburb of Milwaukee."

The nurse nodded. Abruptly, he stopped cleansing my arm, stood tall, and reached again into his deep turquoise pocket. Smiling sheepishly, he pulled out a mini-Snickers bar and unwrapped the candy with a quick, fluid motion. He stuffed the entire chocolate bar in his mouth and chewed voraciously before I could figure out what he was doing. His spittle contained flecks of chocolate and peanuts as he explained, "I need an occasional boost when I work these long twelve-hour shifts."

Andrew and I watched, our mouths agape, when he finally swallowed the candy and returned to my waiting arm.

"I grew up outside the Chicago area," he continued while fumbling with the needle. "Been in Madison for twenty years now, so it feels like home." He placed the tourniquet on my upper arm and flicked my hand with a yellowing fingernail to make the veins appear.

"This sure is a great city for outdoor activities. Even in the winter the die-hards ice fish all day." The nurse droned on until I tuned him out and contemplated what was to come.

The IV was the first step before I would go to the fluoroscopy suite where an interventional radiologist was waiting to place two intracranial electrodes under my temporal lobes. Consequently, in my hospital room, every action would be monitored by camera and the electrical equivalent of my thoughts would be recorded continuously. Even the electrical activity in the deepest parts of my brain would be recorded and monitored and printed on a continuous strip at the front desk of the ward.

As the nurse placed the last piece of tape to secure the IV in place, Andrew's hand rested in a protective position on my back. Next, the nurse wrapped a hospital identification band around my other wrist, securing my position as an inpatient. Then he spun out of the room behind his cart, and an oppressive silence set in as he left. It was official. I was finally walking the path toward epilepsy surgery.

* * *

It wasn't long before another nurse stood in my doorway with a wheelchair and IV pole, waiting to take me down to the procedure center. I attempted to explain that I was perfectly capable of walking down the hall, but the nurse quickly interrupted with an explanation of the V.A.'s rules and regulations. She ushered me into the chair with a huff of satisfaction.

I was nervous about the upcoming procedure, which Dr. Rodgers had warned could be tremendously painful. I attempted a smile when I saw the concern forming on Andrew's face. I searched for a soundtrack to float me into a place of calm. The words to a song that my friend Gretchen, a pastor, wrote circled in my head. "Here I am, Lord, here I am/Here I stand, Lord, here I stand/Let it be with me, let it be." [18]

I sang along silently and felt at peace. *Here I am Lord, these circumstances are beyond my control.* I had to let go of my urge to control, for better or worse, the quality that carried me through my disease and into the good life I cherished. I needed to trust that God would carry me through. A smile grew as I hummed the tune again and again. Perhaps this was my version of Divine Intervention. When I needed a calming hand, I was met with a musical embrace.

The nurse encouraged Andrew to stay behind and wait in my hospital room while she wheeled me to the procedure. Andrew was pleasantly surprised when Emily, a physical therapist at the V.A. and a friend from his childhood, kept him company while I was away. My wheelchair bumped and jangled down the grey hallway until we reached the interventional radiology suite. Eventually I was wheeled into a room that was so painfully stark white and bright I had to avert my eyes. Ahead of me I saw a thin, metal bed in the middle of an enormous donut–shaped machine. I was ushered onto the cold, ominous bed just as the radiology team entered the procedure suite.

The team that joined me in the room included a nurse named Ron, whose extravagant mustache could've made a walrus blush. Jerry, the technician, was himself as large as the fluoroscopy machine. Dr. Ringstad was the radiologist assigned to place the intracranial electrodes. A yellow mask covered her face and rose and fell with each breath. Her sharp green eyes smiled at me to convey comfort and empathy. I squirmed in my metal resting place when Jerry used antiseptic cleanser to sterilize the sides of my face; Ron recorded my blood pressure and vital signs.

Dr. Ringstad felt over my jawline to determine the best location for placement of the electrodes. Her cold fingers crawled like icy spiders from my temples to my ears and she warned me of the importance of staying very still through the entire procedure. After she prepped her materials, Dr. Ringstad nodded to walrus Ron, who floated to the head of the bed and twitched his lips to scratch the tip of his nose with his enormous mustache. Ron placed his vice-like hands on my head and gripped me into a position where I had no choice but to remain still.

"Some patients move involuntarily during this procedure, Kristin," Ron explained. "I'm going to hold tight so you can't flinch or move away." His hands spread in a wide vice from my forehead to my chin and squeezed with force more powerful than my will to move.

I felt Dr. Ringstad's frigid fingers again, then a cold piercing just below my temple. "You're going to feel some pressure now, Kristin," she warned.

Pressure?

The pain was akin to a dentist's drill hitting raw nerve and then pressing deeper, longer, and further. I screamed silently in agony and clenched my teeth in desperation. A metallic taste travelled across my tongue, and a biting shock of pain electrified one side of my face. A single tear traveled down my cheek, and Ron tightened his grip. Once she was satisfied with the placement of the first electrode, Dr. Ringstad asked, "Are you OK?"

All I could do was blink assent. My voice escaped me and Ron's hands prevented me from nodding. After a short pause, Dr.

Ringstad repeated the grueling process on the other side. The entire procedure was finished in about fifteen minutes, and finally Ron and Dr. Ringstad let go.

Ron whispered to his coworkers, "She's a good patient."

Despite the fact that I felt as if there were two holes bored in the side of my face, I was flattered by his compliment.

On the trip back to my hospital room, I leaned into the security of the vinyl wheelchair and gladly accepted the company of the escort who wheeled me back. My head was wrapped in gauze, and EEG wires cascaded from my head. A sharp pain ricocheted from my jaw to my head and back if I attempted to open my mouth even the slightest bit. The short procedure rendered me as vulnerable and as much in need as any of the patients I'd seen on the 8th floor neurology ward.

Soon after I settled back into my colorless hospital room, a nurse plugged the end of my EEG wires into a computer, and I was officially tethered. Gently, she explained that the attached extension cord would give me the "freedom" to cross the room if needed, but it was important that I spend most of my time in the hospital bed. She reminded me that I could unplug briefly to go to the adjacent bathroom, but otherwise the video camera mounted above would record my actions and movements 24/7. She informed me that I should eat in bed while using the small bedside table, though my searing jaw pain made the thought of eating anything objectionable. Finally, she handed me a small hand-held alarm with a white button at the end.

"Press this if you feel a seizure coming," she said. "Someone will be in right away to assist you."

I eyed the device with suspicion. I'd spent so long trying to ignore and ward off the evil beasts that brought the seizures; it was unsettling to hope for one. In order to prove that my seizures originated in the area the neurologists and neurosurgeons proposed to remove, it was important to capture one or more seizures on EEG. I was becoming familiar with irony's closest cousins, hope and desperation.

I settled in and laid my head back on the pillow, tossing and turning in a vain attempt to find a comfortable place to rest between the wires and dressings. I opened my mouth to yawn but stopped halfway when the pain triggered by my intracranial electrodes bolted through my face. Eventually I sank back and fell into a restless sleep, knowing that the clerks at the desk were watching my every move just as a hawk watches a mouse resting contentedly in a field. If an EEG could record nervousness and anticipation, mine would've been overflowing with activity that night.

The icy view of Lake Mendota from the hospital window constantly changed in small ways, disguised by the uniform bed of white and snow. At first glance, I saw a sea of ice with sparsely arranged fishing shacks peppered on the frozen landscape. But as I studied the view throughout the day, I noticed that the fishing huts appeared and disappeared, moving as quickly as the occasional brave skier across the ice. The winter wind whipped up sharply peaked snowdrifts that dissolved before the sun completed its daily trip across the sky. Time was marked by the enormous shadows that rose and fell on the icy canvas as the moon appeared each evening.

Friends, family, and a few colleagues came to visit. Just as when I had the continuous EEG in high school, we coped with my embarrassment and discomfort by laughing at my situation. My friend Shannon gave me a decorative jewel to pin to the front of my gauze turban to make my ominous headdress less foreboding. Maria brought a book on "ways to enrich your brainpower" and challenged me to try the puzzles and mind games and see if there were correlating changes on the EEG. Dr. Isaac stopped by and I immediately transformed from an intelligent adult to a small child begging for relief. My fixed position in the hospital bed left hours for thinking and observing every aspect of my small room and limited view outside. Day after day and hour after hour, I stared at the cords and wires and electrographic tracings… and waited.

By the fifth day of continuous monitoring, I was restless. Or more accurately, I was afraid. I began to doubt the presence of epilepsy at all. Was this all just a big mistake? Were my "seizures" really panic attacks or psychosomatic episodes or nothing at all? Had I put myself and my loved ones through all of this for no reason other than a hyperactive imagination?

I wallowed in doubt and self-pity until I heard a faint knock at my door.

"Mr. Seaborg?" a small voice called from the hallway.

"Uh…yes?" There was little use correcting anyone who called me "Mister" any more.

"May I come in?"

"Of course."

The thick door crept open and revealed a school-aged girl, dressed head-to-toe in Brownie gear and holding a paper sack filled with homemade Valentines. She took a big breath and trained her wide brown eyes on me as she spoke. "On behalf of Brownie Troop 324, I wanted to thank you for your years of service to our country!" She smiled and proudly handed me a glue-heavy construction paper Valentine adorned with stickers, yarn, and uncooked macaroni noodles.

I reached to receive the undeserved recognition and swallowed back my emotional response to the beauty and selflessness of this child. Unbeknownst to her, the simple card directed to the wrong person (Mr. Seaborg was at work) for the wrong reason (I wasn't a veteran) was enough to help me find rays of hope scattered in my puddle of self-pity.

A constant trickle of children visited my room that afternoon to dispense their versions of construction paper gold. I also received a fine-toothed comb, a handkerchief, and a hand-knitted Afghan. Part of me felt guilty for accepting the children's gifts, but I was so lonely and afraid that I couldn't bear to tell them the truth.

Kindness is the most effective antidote to doubt and despair.

* * *

E

Although I wasn't a Veteran, my inpatient stay for video EEG monitoring took place at the VA Hospital because the William S Middleton Veteran's Hospital in Madison is designated an Epilepsy Center of Excellence (ECoE). The ECoE had state-of-the-art video EEG monitoring equipment and the most robust regional inpatient monitoring unit. These services were appreciated by patients like me and imperative for the thousands of veterans returning from conflicts in Iraq and Afghanistan.

Traumatic brain injury (TBI) has been labeled the signature wound of modern day combat due to the proliferation of improvised explosive devices. A study published in the *New England Journal of Medicine* in 2008 showed that nearly 15% of soldiers reported injury consistent with a mild traumatic brain injury after a one-year deployment to Iraq.[19] In 2015, Mary Jo Pugh studied approximately 200,000 soldiers returning from Iraq and Afghanistan and proved that veterans with a history of TBI are 28% more likely to develop epilepsy than those without a history of TBI. Veterans who suffered penetrating brain injury carry the highest risk.

In fact, of the 1.64 million soldiers who've served in Operation Enduring Freedom and Operation Iraqi Freedom, 19% experienced TBI. As many as one third of veterans with moderate to severe TBI and one-half of veterans with penetrating skull injuries developed post-traumatic epilepsy.[20]

Though the numbers are staggering, the full burden of post-traumatic epilepsy from the wars in Iraq and Afghanistan is still not known. A Vietnam Head Injury Study showed that 44% of veterans who experienced penetrating brain injury in the Vietnam War developed post-traumatic epilepsy. However, 14% of these patients didn't experience symptoms until over a decade from time of injury.[21]

18

WITH DR. RODGERS' ENCOURAGEMENT, Andrew planned a
St. Valentine's Day celebration with me in the hospital. He skipped in
like a small child late on Valentine's Day afternoon, arms loaded with
champagne, Bailey's Irish Cream and several DVDs. Alcohol lowered
my seizure threshold, so Andrew brought drinks to invite an event
to end my hospital stay. Sleep deprivation also made seizures more
likely, so we planned to stay up most of the night watching movies.

After I finished my meal of bland mashed potatoes and soup—
the soft food was easier for my sore jaw to tolerate—we found two
plastic cups and squeezed next to each other on the thin hospital bed.

Andrew carefully put his arm around me. I melted into his side
and tried to balance the electrode-free parts of my head on his shoulder. "I love you and I'm proud of you," he said. "No matter what, I'll
always be here for you."

The sincerity etched in the lines on his face made my heart ache.
I knew the hospital stay and expectations of surgery were as stressful to him as to me. "Thank you," I managed, hoping that I could
convey a world of emotion in two simple words. "I love you, too.
Happy Valentine's Day."

We clunked our plastic cups together and giggled at the pecu-
liarity of the setting and our romantic Valentine's Day. We avoided

appearing too affectionate since we knew that a team of nurses watched and recorded my every move. We drank to our marriage and each other through matching mischievous grins.

Later, we watched a grainy version of *Roman Holiday* on the small mounted television while we continued to drink. The video camera brushed aside any fleeting thought of an intimate moment, even when Gregory Peck held princess Audrey in his arms. I was definitely tipsy after three cups of champagne and a small side of Bailey's on ice. Because I didn't usually drink, the sensation of my head spinning and legs wobbling was both foreign and intimidating. If that was what it felt like to be drunk, I decided that I wasn't missing anything.

Andrew left well after midnight as *American President* drew to a close and I was again alone in my hospital cell with its unforgiving white sheets and wires. I slumped back into bed after I switched the DVD to play *Ferris Bueller's Day Off* and was quickly overcome with sleepiness. Only seconds passed before I drifted off to sleep.

That night, I dreamt of smiling Brownies and construction paper Valentines lined in a row, encircling me as I slept, watching and waiting patiently. One by one, the Brownies approached me, singing "Thank you for your years of service to our country." I tried to correct the angelic girls, to tell them that I wasn't worthy of their thanks and didn't deserve their love. My desperation rose as they closed in around me with robotic precision, chanting, *For your country for your country for your county.*

Suddenly, a violent, loud alarm and far-away voices interrupted my dream. I heard a nearby suctioning sound and someone or something pulled my lip. I struggled to open my eyes. There was a hand on my wrist, another on my shoulder. The confusion and muffled noises continued until one voice emerged clearly from the chaos. "Kristin?"

My eyes didn't comply with my wishes to open them. I flinched when two plastic prongs were shoved into my nostrils followed by a *whoosh* of cold air.

"Kristin?"

Unable to open my eyes and wake, I listened to the sounds in the room.

"She's had a grand mal seizure," one voice said. "About seven minutes. She bit her tongue a few times, but the bleeding has stopped. I think she's starting to come around."

Both alarm and relief flared in my subconscious as I drifted back to into milky unconsciousness.

Finally.

* * *

I woke the following morning to muscle pain, a sore mouth and tongue, and an emerging feeling of hope. While the fisherman set up their huts on the icy lake outside, the nurses and residents who visited me on rounds regarded me with a combination of empathy and surprise. After five days of patient waiting, I'd flipped from a peaceful sleep to a generalized seizure in a nanosecond.

Later that morning, the neurology resident stopped in to complete her morning rounds. I knew her both from the previous five days of inpatient monitoring as well as the rotation where we'd worked together in the pediatric neurology clinic months before. She assumed a relaxed position and settled into the rocking chair next to my bedside even though she carried a daunting stack of notes on all the patients she had to see that morning.

"How are you feeling?"

I smiled and mustered a weak smile. "Sore. Tired. But I'm happy I may go home today."

The resident pulled one knee to her chin and gathered her long, black hair into a ponytail. She cocked her head in a gesture of understanding and rocked slowly in the chair. "It's been a long week," she said. "It looks like you celebrated Valentine's Day in style."

I looked at my tongue in the hand-held mirror to find two gouge marks on either side while she talked. There was still blood trickling from the deeper of the two bites.

"That looks painful. Would you like some numbing ointment for your mouth?" she offered.

"No, I'm OK," I said, assuming our visit was over.

Instead of leaving, the neurology resident rested her head on the back of the rocking chair and sat in silence for a while. I wasn't sure if she was resting or just waiting for something else to happen. Eventually, she lifted her head and looked at me through her chestnut eyes.

"Are you ready to go back to work?" she asked. She was intimately familiar with the grueling hours of residency.

"As ready as I'll ever be," I replied. I was anxious to rejoin the world outside my hospital room.

"Take care of yourself, Kristin," she said, while putting a gentle hand on my forearm. "I know none of this is easy. Don't hesitate to reach out if you need a hand on the wards."

She picked up her notes and shuffled out of the room. I watched her leave and reflected on her expression of compassion and encouragement. As the practice of medicine has changed, practitioners are encouraged to be increasingly efficient. There's less time to know a patient beyond their disease. The few extra moments that the neurology resident spent in my bedside chair and the attention she paid to me as a fellow human made all the difference in the world. By quietly challenging the system, she helped me heal.

I resolved to do the same with my patients in the future.

*   *   *

Dr. Rodgers practically skipped into my hospital room wearing a conspicuous smile. "We caught it," he cheered. "The seizure started in your right temporal lobe, exactly where we thought it would. The recordings from your right intracranial electrode really spiked at the beginning of the seizure."

I returned his smile and ignored the dull twinge of pain when I moved my jaw. "Is that enough?" I asked, hopefully. "Can I go home now?"

"Well, we wanted to see more seizures," he ventured, his eyebrows bouncing as he talked. "But that likely won't happen. I know you've had exponentially more sleep and downtime in the hospital than you do normally. I'll take this data to the Epilepsy Conference and see if my colleagues agree that you're a candidate for surgery."

Not completely satisfied, I repeated my question. "Can I go home now?"

I waited the better part of the day for electrode removal, paperwork, and a period of observation after the grand mal seizure. But as the afternoon waned, I finally walked out the confining hospital doors. I devoured the crisp, cold winter air as if I'd been drowning and picked EEG glue out of my hair while Andrew and I walked to the car. I half-expected to hear the mechanical hum of the surveillance camera before I remembered that that chapter of my pre-surgical journey was finally over.

The adage that you don't appreciate something until it's gone is true. After my hospital stay, I was thankful for the mundane comforts that I took for granted: the ability to open my mouth without a jolt of pain, run my hand through my hair, move without an audience, and breathe the frosty February air. No one could tell me what the future would bring, but at that moment I was free. And that was enough.

19

WHEN I SETTLED BACK into my role as a pediatric resident the following week, everything looked different. As a patient, I was surprised by the fear invoked by "quick procedures" and the helplessness induced by "let's wait and see." I had a new understanding of why it was important to avoid swift, robotic patient visits, and why it was my responsibility to offer a comforting hand, spend an extra moment in the bedside chair, or look a patient in the eyes. My experience on the other side of the stethoscope revealed that the little things that make us distinctly human are imperative for success in the long journey toward health.

Although secure in my decision to become a pediatrician, I was still unsure if I wanted to practice general pediatrics or sub-specialize in pediatric neurology. To help with my career choice, I completed my next rotation at the closest hospital with a pediatric neurology training program, the Children's Hospital of Wisconsin. I stayed with my parents at my childhood home in a Milwaukee suburb and traveled to the nearby hospital for the next six weeks. When I moved back into my childhood bedroom in the placid comfort of my parents' home, adult responsibility and reality sloughed off my shoulders for a short, magical time.

During these weeks, I experienced, for the first time, the frustration of the doctors who treat patients with epilepsy. I sat in the corner of the playfully decorated exam rooms and watched a variety of patients, some skipping about with no hint of turmoil inside and some in wheelchairs with drool wetting their shirts. The mystery and cruelty of our common disease was laid starkly before me.

Tyler was born prematurely. He entered the world after twenty-eight weeks gestation instead of the usual forty. Shortly after Tyler was born, he suffered a large intracranial bleed that left him with cerebral palsy, epilepsy, and developmental delay.

At eight years of age, Tyler sat upright yet twisted in his wheelchair with a coat of thick saliva painted on his left cheek, streaming down to his shoulder. When we spoke to him, he offered an inviting smile and looked up with comprehending blue eyes that belied his tortuous muscles and limbs. Tyler was on the maximum allowable dose of the anti-epilepsy medication lamotrigine but he continued to have frequent partial seizures that generalized to grand mal seizures at least once each month.

Tyler's parents were frustrated. His teachers at school were increasingly wary of their ability to care for him with such frequent, violent seizures. For both, the constant fear that he could have a seizure at any moment made it almost impossible for either to attend to the activities and events of their other children, whether siblings or classmates. Caring for Tyler demanded all of their energy.

Dr. Zimmerman, the pediatric neurologist I was working with, sighed when she considered Tyler's situation. He'd been on almost every available anti-epileptic medication without improvement. Several of the previous medications left him so lethargic that he slept through most days. Tyler wasn't a surgical candidate because there was no identifiable focus for his seizures. He was almost out of options.

While Dr. Zimmerman and Tyler's parents talked about the remaining treatment possibilities, I studied the small boy before me. He was dressed in a crisp, yellow polo shirt and pressed khaki pants that were wrinkled only in the small spot where he twisted and pulled the material with his left hand. His dark brown hair crested at the top of his head into a boyish cowlick and his clear blue eyes were the color of a cloudless summer sky. He was a beautiful boy.

Dr. Zimmerman recommended the addition of a small dose of a newer anti-epilepsy medication, levetiracetam, to his other medications. She gave Tyler's parents a prescription for a sedative to use in the event that he had a prolonged seizure. When Tyler's mom wheeled him out of the office, Dr. Zimmerman slumped into her desk.

"These are the hardest ones for me," she explained. "He's so fragile, but I have few other tools to help him." Dr. Zimmerman ran a hand through her hair, stood, straightened her skirt, and marched purposefully to the next exam room. She had no time to dwell on the intractability of her powerlessness.

The scene in the next brightly painted exam room was starkly different. Jennifer was a beautiful, lanky preteen who rested her head against the bright blue wall with an expression of composed indifference. When I introduced myself, Jennifer snapped her gum and fingered her necklace. "Uh, hi."

Dr. Zimmerman summarized Jennifer's pertinent health history. Jennifer developed meningitis after an infection with a community-acquired herpes virus when she was fifteen-months-old. The potent virus attacked Jennifer's temporal lobes and formed a lesion that was invisible on the outside but easily discernible on her MRI. To the innocent bystander, Jennifer appeared the picture of health. Her crisp, cotton dress hung comfortably on her youthful, tan body, and the light danced on slick mahogany hair as if she stood in perpetual sunlight. While her parents updated Dr. Zimmerman on her seizures over the past month, Jennifer fixed her gaze on a magazine which advertised "Cool New Summer 'Dos!" on the cover.

Jennifer's story sounded unnervingly familiar. Her temporal lobe epilepsy had been difficult to control, and she was in the middle of the pre-operative testing for a temporal lobectomy. She was in Dr. Zimmerman's office to review the results of her recent studies and schedule a date for her upcoming epilepsy surgery. Dr. Zimmerman summarized the findings of her recent video EEG monitoring, Wada test, and neuropsychiatric testing. Jennifer continued to exude disinterest as Dr. Zimmerman discussed what she could expect during her post-surgical hospital stay.

I admired Jennifer. I noticed multiple bruises from prior blood tests and procedures splashed on her hands, elbows, and forearms. Her arms hinted at the bruised and battered body beneath.

Dr. Zimmerman gave her a slip of paper with the pediatric neurosurgeon's name and contact information. She offered a heartfelt smile and told Jennifer that the neurosurgery office would contact them soon with a date for surgery. Despite the gravity of upcoming procedure, everyone in the room breathed a sigh of relief. Hope hung thick in the air.

Dr. Zimmerman looked at me with excitement and expectation in her eyes when we finally stepped out of the room. "She's one of the lucky ones," she said. "She has a seizure focus that we can remove, and there's a chance she will be cured."

I watched Dr. Zimmerman disappear down the hall. I couldn't help but wonder if I, like Jennifer, might find a seizure-free existence once the seizure focus was removed. Would I, too, be one of the lucky ones?

* * *

As a second-year pediatric resident who spent up to a hundred hours in the hospital each week, my residency colleagues were much more than co-workers, friends, or fellow trainees. Together, we confronted the grim realities of life and death, sickness, and disease, failure and triumph. We met in the hospital cafeteria at three in the morning and slept next to each other on the dual cracked pink couches in the resident's break room. As the years and the hours slowly marched past, the ties that bound us to each other grew stronger and stronger. In all senses of the word, we were family.

Rarely, there were times when most of us had a free evening. We changed out of our scrubs and met at a colleague's apartment for dinner. Our conversations usually revolved around the craziness of the hospital, which residents were dating whom, and the unusual stories that we encountered every day. For instance, we laughed about the young boy who was tested for cancer before he revealed that his worrisome rash was the result of suctioning a toilet plunger to his chest. We shuddered when we thought about the young girl who fell off her dad's lap while riding the lawn mower and lost an arm and a foot. We hoped we'd never meet another toddler like the one who felt like he had a viral cold one day and died from meningitis the next. Our experiences colored our views of the world. Never again would a lawn mower, plunger, or common cold look the same.

One evening during a jovial post-work dinner, my colleague's husband offered me a glass of wine. By then, I knew that one drink was safe so I happily accepted. My friend's husband, Eric, who was also a physician, looked at me with surprise as I sipped the sweet, cool liquid.

"Are you sure you're OK to drink that, Kristin?" he asked. "You aren't going to do the floppy fish on us, are you?"

Confused, I looked at him for clarification. Instead of explaining more, Eric pulled his arms to his chest in an unnatural, contorted manner and hit his wrists rhythmically against his sternum. He stuck his tongue out and made a yelping sound like a tortured sea lion.

"You know, the floppy fish," he exclaimed, in between arm thrusts and yelps. "A seizure!"

My resident friends snickered and I laughed as well. Although Eric's pantomime was genuinely funny to watch, I couldn't decide whether to be amused or offended by his show. For added effect, Eric twisted his neck and rolled his eyes upwards. He contorted and jived until he'd had enough.

I comforted my friends and colleagues by reporting that I'd had small amounts of alcohol before without untoward effects. One of my perceptive colleagues then took advantage of the silence and quickly changed the subject. Within moments, we were all immersed in a lively conversation about the bulldog-like behavior of the pediatric nephrology attending. Eric caught my eye and threw me a winning smile. Warily, I smiled back.

I wasn't sure why I was bothered by Eric's "floppy fish" dance, but I felt unsettled deep within. Perhaps it was as simple as the fact that the entire room had a good laugh at my expense. More likely than that, though, was that the simple joke pointed out my weakness in a room full of physicians. Eric called attention to the fact that, in many ways, I was simply a fish out of water.

Furthermore, I was disturbed that a group of adults with advanced medical training still felt that seizures and epilepsy were a joke. The reality of my everyday fears was far from amusing. The truth of my upcoming surgery left little room for comic relief. If I were ever to change the stigma associated with epilepsy at all, I would have to start with the very doctors who cared for us, the providers who harbored the knowledge and empathy that we needed most.

20

THE WADA TEST was the next step in my pre-surgical testing; a test designed to determine the location of language and short-term memory in my brain. Dr. Rodger's nurse gently explained that during the test, a radiologist would insert a catheter into the large femoral artery in my groin and push the catheter through my arterial system until it was in position to inject a sedative into the carotid arteries in my neck. When the sedative was infused into one carotid artery at a time, it would anesthetize one side of my brain for five to ten minutes. While I was awake with half of my brain anesthetized, a neuropsychologist would show me a variety of objects to see if I could access the memory and language to name them. Simple enough, right?

I was terrified.

On the day of the Wada test, I walked into UW hospital with my mother and tried to ignore the lump of anxiety that occupied the pit of my stomach. My mom eagerly filled in the role of supportive family member while Andrew was in Japan on business. Just as during the trip to Mayo four years before, it was a tremendous comfort to have her with me.

We traversed the immense, rotating doors to enter the same hospital where I was a resident physician twelve hours earlier. My life as a physician/patient felt as if I was constantly rotating from one role to another, just as the automatic revolving door ushered patients across the threshold between vulnerable and independent. At the patient registration desk, the man behind the counter strapped a hospital band to my wrist and my transformation was again complete.

Later that morning, I waited half-dressed underneath a thin white sheet in the long hall outside the procedure room. My mom stood at attention by my side and gripped the guardrails on my bed until her knuckles blanched as white as my insufficient covering. The interventional radiologist stopped to visit in between procedures to explain her role and obtain my consent for the Wada test.

She began to talk in layman's terms. "I will use a catheter, or a long tube, starting in this artery in your groin." She pointed to the location where the femoral artery travels across the crease between upper leg and pelvis. "Once in place, I'll snake the catheter all the way up to the big artery in your neck." She pointed to the location of the carotid artery.

I nodded like a diligent student and murmured assent while she explained what to expect. She moved on to explain the risks of the procedure.

My mother, who continued to grip and un-grip the gurney's side rails, finally gave in to her maternal pride. In the middle of a basic explanation of another risk, Mom blurted, "You know, Kristin is a doctor."

I slipped back through the figurative revolving doors. The radiologist looked at me again and tried to find where the M.D. was hidden underneath my thin sheet of exposure.

"Really?" she asked. "What kind?"

"I'm a second year pediatrics resident," I explained. My face burned with embarrassment. Although only eighteen months out of medical school, I was ingrained enough in the medical culture that I believed physicians themselves weren't supposed to have illnesses — especially illnesses that may interfere with cognitive function.

To my relief, the radiologist paused for only a fleeting moment before regaining her composure. She resumed her explanation in technical terms. The discussion of anatomy and biochemistry of the Wada test was surprisingly reassuring.

Finally, I signed the consent paperwork and Mom unwrapped her protective fists. The radiologist wheeled my bed around the corner into yet another sterile room and the test began.

Despite my worry, the Wada test was uneventful. The radiologist took a moment to point out my cerebral vessels on the fluoroscopy screen since she knew I learned the anatomy in medical school. I don't remember large portions of the procedure after the initial injection of dye and anesthetic. I remember being asked to hold my hands straight forward and identify a plastic chair and a miniature bike. I remember when I was wheeled back down the cold hall to the recovery room, where my mom patiently waited. I remember the persistent dull throb over the site in my groin where a long, thin needle was inserted to access my femoral artery.

When I read the procedure report afterwards, I learned that there was a long period when I couldn't speak after the left side of my brain was anesthetized. I had very little short-term memory when I was forced to use my compromised right hemisphere alone, presumably because of the permanent damage to brain structures that occurred during my first seizure.

The results were both encouraging and unsettling. The Wada test proved that the portion of my brain that controls language was in the left hemisphere. My prolonged seizure as a toddler forced my malleable immature circuitry to re-wire most of my short-term memory to my left temporal lobe. All of the diagnostic tests confirmed that my right temporal lobe was the source of my seizures but had little beneficial function.

I was officially a surgical candidate.

*   *   *

I worked with the neurosurgery team and my pediatric residency director to schedule surgery at a time when I wouldn't fall behind in my expected residency duties. After careful consideration, we scheduled surgery in mid-May, thereby taking advantage of the small amount of time that residents have before the start of the new academic year on July 1st.

After my six weeks of pediatric neurology at Children's Hospital in Milwaukee, the last rotation I completed in the weeks before surgery was pediatric cardiology at UW Hospital. I was assigned to participate in surgeries to repair small defects in children's hearts during the first part of the rotation. My own surgery loomed ominously, so I paid close attention to the atmosphere in the operating room before, during, and after each procedure. I found that the pre-operative period was an especially scary time for the patients—trembling children, really—who rolled into the large, cold O.R. to meet a sea of faceless doctors hidden behind masks, gowns, and hairnets.

I smiled at these children and used my unmasked eyes to offer comfort, but my profile was only one of many in the room full of strangers. When the anesthesiologist asked each child to scoot from the padded gurney to the unforgiving metal bed, I squeezed reassurance in my lifting hand. I hoped that my efforts to make the O.R. even slightly less frightening for these children would be repaid by similarly motivated well-wishers when it was my turn to lie underneath the scalpel and lights.

I was surprised by the amount of conversation and banter in the O.R. throughout every procedure. Over a child's open chest, the attending surgeon chatted with a resident about the upcoming Farmer's Market. When the physicians were wrist-deep in warm blood and a tangle of vital vessels, the nurses answered pages, gave updates to families, and shared anecdotes about their own families. When the procedures were finished and the wounds closed, the entire surgical team waited patiently while each child woke from their drug-induced sleep.

It was especially difficult to watch the children emerge from anesthesia when their indwelling breathing tubes impeded the innate instinct to breathe. The small waking patients bucked and coughed with monumental force and attempted to purge the tubes before the anesthesiologist removed them. I hoped that the children, and I, wouldn't remember the frightful sensation of plastic corking each breath.

I joined the medical team to walk each fresh post-operative patient to the safety of the Post-Anesthesia Care Unit (PACU). The general pediatric inpatient ward was situated immediately between the operating rooms and the PACU. Time after time throughout each day, the staff on the pediatric ward watched a succession of patients stripped of clothes, consciousness, and dignity. I made a mental note to request that when my turn came, the transporting team take a route that wouldn't pass the pediatric patients and staff. I couldn't let my colleagues and coworkers see me that way.

I completed a different part of my pediatric cardiology rotation the week before my surgery. I worked in the outpatient pediatric cardiology clinic with Dr. Sadma while she read echocardiograms. I observed her quietly from the corner of a dark room and learned about pediatric structural heart defects from fuzzy grey images of the heart pulsating on the television screen. One morning I was struggling to stay awake when my pager beeped with an unfamiliar number. I roused from my corner in the dark conference room to answer.

"Hi, this is Kristin Seaborg returning a page."

"Oh, hi, Kristin. It's Sarah from Dr. Isaac's office." In one sentence, Dr. Isaac's nurse practitioner had seamlessly morphed me again from doctor to patient. "I was wondering if you were planning on donating your own blood for your surgery."

My pulse increased as I furtively studied the dimly lit conference room. I wasn't ready for anyone else to hear this conversation. I snuck around to a far corner and responded quietly and quickly. "I can't because the last time I donated blood I had a grand mal seizure." I waited for nearby doctors to look up, but no one heard me.

"What?" Sarah sounded puzzled on the other end of the line.

I repeated in a hushed voice, "No. Giving blood makes me have seizures."

"I'm sorry, Kristin, I can't hear you."

Exasperated and embarrassed, I kept my final answer succinct. "No!"

I scanned the room again. Dr. Sadma was still reading echocardiograms, unaware of my frustration or even my presence. My continued level of discomfort surprised me. More than half of the pediatric attending doctors knew that I was having brain surgery within a few days, but I was still too embarrassed to utter the word "seizure" without feeling ashamed.

I fumbled my way back to my observation chair next to Dr. Sadma, thankful that the darkness in the room hid my face. I feigned interest in the grey-scale images and swallowed back my unease.

Who was I? Did I even belong here? Could I be both a doctor and a patient at the same time without sinking in humiliation or floating only in illusions? I was a chameleon who changed the color of my outer coat depending on my surroundings. I prayed that I wouldn't have to run and hide for much longer.

21

THE EVENING BEFORE my surgery, I took a long walk and hoped that nature and warming spring air would still my brewing nervousness. In the sweet smelling dusk, the world burst with the promise of spring. The waking tree branches hung low, heavy and swollen with emerging buds.

My thoughts fell in cadence with the rhythm of my brisk walk. I repeated the same phrase again and again as my feet pounded the pavement like a metronome. *The hard part is over, all I have to do is show up. The hard part is over, all I have to do is show up. The hard part is over, all I have to do is show up. . .*

The stress of medication changes, diagnostic tests, and waiting for surgery while working eighty to one hundred hours a week had been incredibly challenging. The assignment to show up at the hospital early and let Dr. Isaac take over was comparatively simple.

The birds chirped a reassuring evening song. As always, the beauty of my surroundings grounded me. I arrived home serene and expectant.

Andrew immediately noticed the difference. "Are you O.K.?"

"Yes." My response surprised him. "I just need to organize my suitcase for tomorrow."

I padded down the hallway to our bedroom and packed for a several-day hospital stay. I folded my flannel cat pajamas and carefully placed them next to several pairs of underwear, slippers, and multiple dog-eared books. Later, I showered and washed thoroughly using the antiseptic solution Hibiclens, as instructed by Dr. Isaac's nurse. The pungent orange solution's distinct smell immediately conjured images of the hospital and operating rooms. I wondered how long it would be before I could independently take a hot shower again.

I slowly brushed my hair and studied my profile in the mirror. My thick, dark hair moved in the light and the shadows danced on my long face. I smiled at my reflection and found the beginnings of faint wrinkles hidden along the outside corner of my eyes. I studied my untamed eyebrows and prominent nose (passed down through the generations on my father's side) and wondered how surgery might change the contour of my face. Dr. Isaac assured me that he would shave only a small amount of hair, but I was doubtful about what would remain. I wondered if the titanium plate used to close my skull would alter the outline of my silhouette or if the eventual scar on my head would leave an obvious mark that announced my epilepsy.

There was nothing left to do after I was packed, scrubbed, and organized. I was used to having a perpetual to-do list, so the absence of responsibilities unnerved me. I finally surrendered and climbed into our warm bed after hours of needless fussing. Andrew, hoping to convey comfort and affection, immediately sidled next to me and gathered me in his arms. I struggled to say the things that'd been lingering on my mind for days.

"I have two things to tell you," I ventured. I wanted to get this right.

"Anything, Kristin," he whispered into my ear.

"Full code," I croaked. It may've been a bit melodramatic, but I wanted to make sure that Andrew knew I wished for a full resuscitation should anything disastrous happen in the O.R.

"Of course." Andrew's face fought to find the middle ground between bemusement and concern. "What else?"

I took another deep breath, "Organ donor." I hid the tears that sprung to my eyes but my husband heard the fear in my wavering voice. Still, it was important that he knew I would donate my organs to others if catastrophe struck.

"Don't worry, Kristin. I'm here." He paused. "Are you scared?"

"No," I lied. "Just nervous."

Andrew didn't pester me to define the difference between "scared" and "nervous" and I didn't elaborate on the whirlwind of thoughts running through my head. Instead, I rested in his arms and surrendered my barricade of stoicism. Finally, I accepted that it was all right to lean on my husband and my family through my most frightening hours. There was no turning back and I needed to trust that I made the right decision to proceed with surgery.

When morning arrived, I would have a hole drilled in my head and a sizable portion of my brain removed. In the comfort of my bed that evening, I closed my eyes and rested with confidence and hope that everything would go as planned. I imagined that no one would take a leap of faith if they knew the full truth of what was on the other side.

*   *   *

The sky blushed with expectation when Andrew and I drove to the hospital just after 6 A.M. the following morning. We shuffled in our pre-caffeinated state to the surgical floor and through the door of the First Day Surgery Suite.

A chipper nurse greeted us and ushered me into a small stall surrounded by curtains. She ordered me to undress and change into a thin, shapeless hospital gown. Again thinly covered and defenseless, I remembered my recent admissions for the inpatient EEG, Wada test, and PET scan. I was begrudgingly familiar with the sensation of being powerless.

This time, however, was different. Within a few hours, Dr. Isaac and his team would have the opportunity to literally pick my brain. No one knew what the day would reveal.

Andrew and I pretended to watch the morning edition of CNN on the small mounted television while he shifted uncomfortably in his bedside seat and clenched my hand. We were too anxious to talk, so he did his best by rubbing my knee and sent amorous glances my way. When one of the curtains moved, I looked up and expected to see Dr. Isaac. Instead, I was thrilled to meet the warm smile of one of our dear friends and pastors, Peter.

Peter sat on the corner of my bed and enveloped my non-occupied hand. "How are you doing?" he asked affectionately.

"OK," I said. Peter knew I wasn't telling the truth.

"I know you don't have long before you go, but I'm here to say hello and say a prayer with you and Andrew," he explained. Peter reached his other hand to grip Andrew's and bowed his head.

He prayed for my strength and safety, for Andrew's fortitude and endurance, and for the skills of the surgeons' hands. Later, Peter sat with Andrew, Andrew's parents, and mine, and waited through my marathon seven-hour surgery. For all of us, Peter's comforting presence stands out as one of the things that made a practically unbearable day achievable.

Almost immediately after Peter left my curtained enclosure for the surgical waiting room, Dr. Isaac and the anesthesiology resident stopped by. I shrunk a few millimeters into my white sheet when I recognized Mike, the anesthesiology resident assigned to my case. Mike was a medical school classmate and distant friend. He tried to hide his recognition and surprise and reassume a professional demeanor.

Mike ambled tentatively up to my bedside and offered a crooked half-smile. At seven in the morning, his blue scrubs already looked as if they had a few days of living in them. The front of his shirt had a linear drip line of coffee down the middle and scattered grease stains from an early breakfast. His hospital-issued pants were bunched up and cinched tightly in the middle in attempt to counteract the weight of his pagers pulling them down. I sensed Mike's discomfort but he graciously stepped closer to rest his hand on my shoulder.

"Hey, Kristin. Funny to meet you here." Mike crumpled his words so that they came out bunched and uneven, just like his scrubs.

"Kinda weird, isn't it?" I offered. "Wasn't it it just last week when we were in the O.R. together with that ASD repair?"

Mike laughed. "Yeah. Now it's your turn."

I managed a nervous chuckle at the irony of my situation. "Are you here to place my IV?" I asked.

"Yes. I also need to do a quick exam." With an air of formality, Mike searched for the radial pulses in my wrists, listened to my heart and lungs, and examined my head and neck. He explained that he would put in an IV in the pre-op area, but would place more permanent access in my radial artery once I was asleep. With the consult over, we made small talk for a few minutes before Mike leaned back and looked from Andrew to me. "Well, it's time to get going. I have some midazolam to calm your nerves before we bring you down to the operating room. Midazolam may also cause short-term amnesia so you won't remember much after we give you the medication." He paused. "Now would be a good time to say goodbye."

I was already drunk with apprehension but dutifully leaned over and clasped Andrew's hand while Mike injected the medication into my IV. Andrew's presence reassured me, and I leaned back into my bed to rest.

That's all I remember from the pre-operative period. The next thing I can recall is my abrupt return to consciousness immediately after surgery. Andrew told me later that I continued to talk with him and became progressively loopy until Mike determined it was time to wheel me down the long hallway to the operating suites. Andrew said that as my gurney turned the corner and slipped from view, I gave one last loud, raucous laugh as though I was responding to someone's joke. I like to think that I was laughing in the face of epilepsy.

* * *

E

Temporal lobe epilepsy (TLE) is the most common form of focal, or partial, epilepsy. Those with TLE also represent the largest group of patients with treatment-resistant epilepsy.[22] Although anti-epileptic medications are effective for two-thirds of patients with temporal lobe epilepsy, up to one

third of patients are burdened with medication-resistant temporal lobe seizures.

Just as in my case, surgical resection of a
seizure focus is an option for treatment in some
patients with documented hippocampal changes on
MRI. Although surgery offers the best chance that
many TLE patients have for a cure, longitudinal
studies have shown that although many patients
achieve a reduction in their seizures, fewer attain
a true cure.

When I first considered surgery in 1996, I was
told that temporal lobe surgery held a 95% chance
of reduction or resolution of my seizures. By the
time I rolled down the hallway to the O.R. in 2003,
I knew the current data revealed that only 50% of
TLE patients were rendered seizure-free ten years
after temporal lobectomy.[23] It was a chance I was
willing to take.

22

WATER.

A long stream of water flowed down my trachea, and my motionless lips tried in vain to grapple for air. I flailed in a sea of breathless unconsciousness before I heard a loud suction sound as if a large suckerfish was removed from my throat. I managed several thirsty breaths on my own before I drifted back to the black sea of unconsciousness.

One by one, a variety of voices drifted into my sphere of understanding. A collection of hands crawled like spiders under and around me and attached and detached stickers and probes to every uncovered surface of my body. Limp and lifeless as a rag doll, nameless hands tilted me sideways and back onto a straight board.

"On my count," one of the voices called. "One...two...three!"

The hammock of collective hands lifted me from the cold surgical bed and deposited me on a new gurney. I couldn't talk, but I was able to slowly take a blind inventory of my surroundings. *The surgery must be over*, I thought. With this subconscious realization, I acknowledged a new searing pain in my head and a developing ache all over.

Blackness returned. Time elapsed in my infinite continuum of darkness before the dancing voices trickled back into my foggy awareness. It felt like I was floating on my back in a rough sea when the gurney moved carefully out of the operating suite. A high-pitched voice called above me: "Careful over the bumps! Careful over the bumps!" The lights from one fluorescent bank of lights after another flashed underneath my swollen eyelids like one-toned fireworks. I struggled to understand where I was.

Eventually, the gurney stopped, and I was in another room surrounded by a new chorus of voices. A multitude of hands touched and prodded all over again while they attached blood pressure cuffs, leg stockings, intravenous tubing, and oxygen monitors. A new voice beckoned, "Kristin! Can you open your eyes for me? Kristin?"

I wanted to respond but I could croak nothing but ragged breath. I mustered all my strength to open my small eye-slits that were partially encumbered by dressings and swelling. Dr. Isaac informed me of my post-surgical destination before my surgery. I must've arrived in the Neurosurgical Intensive Care Unit.

"Open your eyes, Kristin!" My new nurse was like a drill sergeant. "I need to wash your face," she explained. "Would you like me to use a cool washcloth or a warm one?"

"Cool," I whispered, struggling to stay awake.

I barely heard the sounds she made as she checked my vital signs and recorded data.

"Kristin!" I was jolted out of my anesthetic-induced slumber. "Open your eyes as wide as you can! Do you want a warm washcloth or a cool one?"

"Cool," I uttered again.

"I can't hear you, honey!" My nurse thought that if she screamed at me I would talk louder. "Warm or cool?"

Irritation and a shattering headache fueled my barely-louder-than-a-whisper final answer. "Cool."

Finally. A cool washcloth gently wiped away what must've been dried blood and mucus from my face and hairline. She rearranged my gauze turban so the dressings didn't overlap my eyes. When she used a wet swab to clean my mouth, I savored the first drips of water offered after the seven-hour surgery.

"It's not time to drink yet, Kristin," she scolded. "This is only to clean your mouth. Let's try again."

A small sponge was pushed into my mouth again. I clenched and sucked as much fluid as I could muster. Usually compliant, my post-operative confidence was bolstered by my small act of defiance. "No, Kristin, it's not time to drink!" she scolded in frustration.

Spent, I fell back into a leaden sleep. An unknown epoch of time passed before I roused again. "Are you in pain?" My nurse had a kinder tone now that she'd completed the face-washing task. I tried to nod without success. "Your blood pressure is high," she said mostly to herself. "I'm going to give you a little morphine to help with the pain." I heard a faint beep and waited for the sensation of a sharp knife in my skull to lessen to a pulsating throb.

Eventually a new, and familiar, voice caressed my ear. "Kristin," Andrew whispered. "Kristin, you're okay. I'm here." One of his hands rested on my leg and the other freed a stray wisp of hair that stuck to my cheek. He sniffed and stood next to me. Was he crying?

"Do you know the last time she stooled?" My nurse still focused on completing her post-operative assessment.

Andrew faltered, "Uh, I have no idea. That's not something we usually talk about." I sensed his nervous smile.

"Do you think it was this morning?" the nurse pressed.

"Could've been, but, uh, I really don't know."

I listened to their conversation until I couldn't stand it anymore. Really? My pooping habits?

I willed my eyes open and summoned the strength to break in.

"Yess-tur-dahy," I muddled. Proud of myself, I chuckled in victory before a new pain jackknifed through my head.

Andrew and my nurse gasped with pleasant surprise—the nurse because she got her answer, Andrew because my one-word response confirmed that I could talk, smile, and understand without my right temporal lobe. A cloud of relief filled the room and I crossed the chasm back into the void of oblivion.

Minutes or hours passed before I recognized two warm hands patting my cheeks. The architecture of the hands conjured a primal source of comfort and familiarity. My mother stood at the head of my bed.

I heard her talk to the nurse and listened as if I were in another room.

"What are these?" Mom asked. "Why does she have these things on her legs?"

"Those are compression stockings," the nurse explained. "They inflate and deflate to make sure Kristin doesn't develop a blood clot while she's lying still in bed."

"And what's this thing on her finger? Why does she have this?"

I wanted to explain, *It's a pulse ox, Mom. It measures the level of oxygen in your blood. Everyone has one of these after surgery.* But my ability to speak had again vanished.

I listened silently and motionlessly while Mom deconstructed every monitor and tube and learned why each one was at my bedside. All the while, her warm hands patted my cheeks and calmed the helpless little girl who lay before her.

The evening crept on with long periods of sleep and pain peppered by a parade of faces. My dad came quietly, as he always did, and offered his encouragement and love with a gentle pat on the arm and a prolonged gaze into my eye-slits. My brother, Jon, appeared at my knee and tentatively asked how I was feeling. His visit was short, but I knew he'd worked behind the scenes for weeks to ensure I had the best possible O.R. staff present during surgery. Dr. Isaac rested a hand on my shoulder and told me the surgery went smoothly. I'm not sure if my garbled reply adequately portrayed my gratitude for his expertise and reassurance.

Later, I learned that the goal-oriented nurse with drill-sergeant qualities sat calmly with Andrew and held his hand through the afternoon and evening while he lingered at my bedside. Jason, the neurosurgery resident who participated in my surgery, left a vase of fresh flowers that transformed a colorless corner of my room.

Jason and my nurse were two more shining examples of those who took steps beyond their area of expertise to practice the art and heart of medicine. Their actions taught me that success as a health care provider doesn't always come from textbooks or scholarly articles, but by looking beyond disease into a hurting soul.

* * *

The day after surgery was a day of elimination. The arterial line, urinary catheter, and leg compression stockings were all removed. My nurse enthusiastically changed and removed my bloody and sweaty head bandage. I was taken off the census of the neurosurgical ICU before my lunch tray arrived.

I felt at home on the general neurology floor. The familiar routine of groups of residents and students marching in and out of my room during daily rounds was reassuring. I took comfort in the predictable daily blood draws, measurement of vital signs, and nursing shift changes. For the first few days after surgery, the landscape of my mundane hospital room was speckled with the friendly faces of well-wishers and friends.

Nancy was my new nurse on the general neurology floor. She wore half-moon pink glasses that slipped repeatedly to the very end of her sharply pointed nose to reveal her coffee-brown eyes. Although she spoke in a kinder tone than that of my nurse the night before, she harbored the same no-nonsense mentality.

"All right, Kristin," she chirped. "It's time for you to get up."

Her command startled me since less than 24 hours had passed since surgery. Before I could protest, she grabbed my arm at the elbow, leaned her large frame into mine and pulled. My feet found the ground and my knees locked into place with trepidation. As soon as I was upright, the ground undulated beneath my feet.

"Whoa!" I gasped when I fell back into bed, gripping my head. "I'm dizzy!"

Undeterred, Nancy gripped my elbow again. "OK, we'll take it slower this time. You can do this."

When my pink-stockinged feet were again on the ground, Nancy carefully guided me into a vertical position. My defiant legs wobbled unsteadily.

"I...can't...find...my...equilibrium," I grunted through clenched teeth. I grappled for a sure stance as beads of sweat accumulated on my forehead. Nancy held tight until I wasn't swaying any more.

"Take a deep breath, Kristin. I've got you. When you're ready, I'm going to let go and let you stand on your own."

My head was pounding. "Ready."

Nancy stayed immediately in front of me but let go of my elbows. Instantly, I sank. Thankfully, Nurse Nancy grabbed me just before I toppled to the ground and firmly guided me back to bed. "We'll try that again later today," she said with a straight glance down her ski-slope nose. "You're still recovering."

The following morning Nancy waited impatiently by my bedside while I finished a few bites of breakfast. "It's a new day," she cheered. "Time to get you moving!"

After analyzing my failure to stand the day before, I knew what was missing. I needed strength, a wide-based stance, and the confidence that I could stay upright. Even overnight, I notably improved in all of these areas.

Nancy let me call the shots so I would feel confident and in control. I grasped her vice-like hand and made the transition from sitting to standing. I stood with effort and sighed with relief when I raised my head to join Nancy in her smile. Within seconds, however, the sinking feeling returned, and I reeled backwards. Nancy caught me quickly and righted my drunken body. So far, at least, balance was beyond my reach. I mentally added this to my running list of things that'd slipped out of my control.

Late the following evening, I lay awake watching reruns of *Friends* when Jason appeared at my door. A neurosurgery resident who'd earned the nickname "Mighty Mouse" because of his modest stature, Jason was only a bit taller than me, but the width of his shoulders and biceps was enough to rival professional body-builders. He spoke in a clipped, purposeful manner that reflected a neurosurgeon's confidence. Jason intimidated most of the medical students and residents in the hospital, but I knew better. In addition to the flowers he brought to the ICU immediately after my surgery, he oversaw the group of residents that rounded on me daily. He'd heard I was having trouble walking and made it his mission to get me better.

"Hey, Kristin!" he quipped from my doorway. "What're you doing lying around? It's time to get up!"

I couldn't help but roll my eyes at his ridiculous request. Before I could protest, a beefy arm encircled my right elbow and lifted my limp body through the air. I was on my feet but my legs refused to comply with my internal command to remain upright. I faltered and expected to be set back down atop the reassuring nest of white hospital sheets again, but Jason wouldn't let go.

"We're going for a walk," he proclaimed. A childish smile travelled across his face. "We've got to get you strong."

I held tightly onto Jason's strong arm and let my fears wash away as we walked. Slowly, the spinning resolved and all the earlier unsteadiness disappeared. I listened as Jason told me in general terms about some of the patients he'd seen in the Emergency Department that evening. My mind relaxed and moved on to things beyond my present broken self. By the time we were on our second lap around the neurology ward, it felt as if I were taking an afternoon stroll with a friend instead of fighting the gravity of my wayward legs.

BEEP! BEEP! BEEP!

The harsh sound of Jason's pager interrupted my thoughts and jolted me back to reality. There was a long, stark hall ahead before I could return to my room and Jason needed to find a phone quickly to answer his page. When we picked up the pace, my knees buckled but Jason still held me fast. "I've got to go back downstairs," he said. "But this isn't the end of our training. I'm on call so I'll be back later tonight or tomorrow to work on getting you back to yourself."

We turned the corner into my room and Jason helped me back into my bed of safety. My head screamed from the effort, but my smile was so wide I may've loosened some of my staples with the pull of my cheeks.

"That was good work," Jason cheered and shook my hand. "Now get some rest so you'll be ready when I come back."

He slid out the door, his white coat dangling on a finger over his shoulder. Alone again, I pressed the pulsing side of my head and slipped further into bed. I fell immediately into a deep, restful sleep.

Jason's visit was the turning point in my hospital stay. He helped me find the confidence to walk on my own while demonstrating what it means to be a good physician. He showed me that a patient is more than their disease. Our frustrations, fears, worries, and dreams all contribute to the cluster of healing and the magic of being well.

I sipped my coffee the next morning while I waited for the parade of rounding teams and thought how the little things leave the most lasting impression. I was appreciative of all the physicians who participated in my care, but I'll always remember the ones who offered compassion and encouragement along the way. I promised myself that when I eventually returned to my doctor role, I would never forget the lessons I learned through the eyes of a patient.

Finally, six days after surgery, it was time to go home. With effort, I demonstrated that I could walk down the hall and upstairs with the assistance of a walker and I was "cleared" by the physical therapist. I was filled with nervous energy on the morning of my hospital discharge. Although excited to return to the comforts of home, I was scared that I would fail without the safety net of doctors, nurses, pharmacists, and other medical staff who'd been constantly present to ensure my safety and recovery.

Andrew and I packed up the flowers, cards, and keepsakes that friends sent with well wishes. He ran back and forth to the car to load the treasures as if he were a cross between a florist and a pack mule. I changed into clean clothes and the nurses removed my IV and cleaned the question mark-shaped surgical wound on the right side of my head for a final time. I sloughed off my patient identity as quickly as I removed my hospital gown and cut my hospital band in a last, victorious, symbolic gesture. Since I was still unable to walk securely, Andrew offered comfort when he wheeled me down the hall through the ward that'd seen my pain, frustration, and recovery. When we entered the elevator and watched the thick doors close behind us, I shut my eyes and hoped that this time I'd truly left seizures behind.

23

I RETURNED HOME from surgery in late May with a walker to use at all times until I was steadier on my feet. In addition to my two usual anti-epileptic drugs, Dr. Rodgers added gabapentin to quell the grueling daily post-operative headaches. I planned to take four to six weeks off for recovery. During the early days back at home, I wasn't sure how I'd return to residency at all.

Only time would tell if the surgery cured my epilepsy. The longer I went without seizures, the more favorable my prognosis. The lengthening days and warming air thawed the frozen ground and renewed my weary spirit. The tissue pathology examination of my resected brain tissue confirmed that my right hippocampus was severely withered and scarred. As the days marched on, it appeared that the neurosurgery team had removed the focal point of my seizures. I continued to take weighty doses of anti-epileptic medications but studied the bottles every morning and hoped that someday they might not be part of my life.

My friends and family visited and called, but the long, lonely days made me feel isolated. Everyone was so careful around me. When Andrew's parents came, they tiptoed tentatively around the condo and talked in hushed tones, careful not to trigger a head-ache. When my resident colleagues dropped by with flowers and a meal, they made sure that their feet were widely planted before they offered a hug so they wouldn't disrupt my fleeting balance. Andrew remained upbeat, chipper, and almost unnaturally positive at all times to prevent a sour mood.

I gradually rebuilt my armor of forced contentment and impenetrable stoicism in effort not to disappoint my friends and family. If I wanted my loved ones to stop acting like I was a ticking time bomb, I had to smile more, sleep less, and grab for fewer railings. My unmasked body and soul would find the time to heal on their own.

A little over a week after I was discharged from the hospital, I was ready to venture outside the protection of my home. The Madison chapter of Pediatricians Recognizing Individuals Demonstrating Excellence (PRIDE) presented its first recognition award to a middle school student.

The summer before my surgery, my friends Julian, Shannon, and I sat at a weathered orange table at the legendary Memorial Union terrace and talked about how we could locally reproduce a program started at the University of Kansas. PRIDE was the brainchild of pediatric residents who wanted to promote positive behaviors in impoverished kids and encourage them to continue down the right path.

In the months after our initial meeting, we asked schools for nominations of outstanding students, solicited businesses for rewards to give the children, and determined the logistics of how we would recognize a new student each month. Finally, we planned to present our first award to an eighth grade student just ten days after my surgery. Although I had trouble walking and standing independently, I wasn't willing to miss the inaugural PRIDE presentation.

Our honoree was a hopeful twelve-year-old boy with dark brown eyes and a quick smile. He lived with his mother and two sisters in a series of temporary residences: first a trailer, then a hotel room, then the bed of a truck parked in various parking lots at night. Despite the obvious hardships, he went out of his way to help others at school. He weeded the school garden on Saturdays, walked a disabled classmate to class, and served in student government.

We planned a big party at a local park for our first PRIDE presentation. We invited the young man's teachers, classmates, family, and all the pediatric residents. Andrew parked as close as he could to the park shelter and offered his arm for support. I held him tightly while we stumbled up the small hill to join the growing crowd. When we shuffled up to the open cooler and dug for a soda, a ripple of recognition travelled through the group.

"Hi, Kristin, it's really nice to see you," our chief resident, Brady, said as he stepped from his spot next to the grill.

"Hey, Kristin! How're you feeling?" Julian called from behind the chip bowl.

"Kristin! So good to see you!" Dave, our residency program director, shouted from the other side of the shelter.

One by one, friends and colleagues offered greetings and an arm of support. My legs were weak and my head pounded, but the warm ring of friendship overpowered my physical complaints. If our honoree could learn kindness and generosity from the back of a pickup, I could learn resilience and humility through pain and dizziness.

I was deeply grateful for the affection and support my resident colleagues offered throughout my illness and surgery. Maria was ever-present for a sympathetic ear or a needed hug. Shannon always offered a helping hand and helped me laugh at myself. Julian was an expert at providing both comic relief and watching my back. We cared for the same struggling patients in the hospital by day and shared the same feelings of inadequacy and frustration at night.

The picture taken at the end of the PRIDE picnic shows a gaggle of smiling pediatric residents and middle school students huddled around a huge homemade banner with *Pediatricians Recognizing Individuals Demonstrating Excellence* painted in large red letters. I'm standing along the edge of the banner, smiling cautiously through clenched teeth. If you look closely, you can see Julian and Brady's protective arms gripping my elbows on both sides to ensure that I wouldn't fall. The smiling children around us are oblivious to the quiet drama of my struggle to remain standing.

The picture is one of recovery. My hair is disheveled, my expression one of concealed discomfort, but I'm held up by those who cared enough to stand near. It was a wonderful day. When my colleagues walked me back to the car to go home, I knew with certainty that I would be just fine.

*   *   *

In the weeks that followed, a new energy blossomed as the crocuses bloomed. The persistent headaches and dizziness retreated as quickly as they came. I returned to work six weeks after I left the same building as an inpatient. My white coat and stethoscope shielded me from the illness that once held me hostage. I walked the pediatric wards as if I'd never left but still paused for a moment when I passed the fork in the hall that led to the neurology ward. When the hospital was quiet, I stood at the end of the pediatric corridor and watched the patients shuffling down the hall on the neurology unit. Hidden in an empty doorway, I was a barely visible, and tentative, observer.

I knew that it was simply a combination of luck and tenaciousness that permitted me to stand again on the other side of the medical construct. I was fortunate to have a discernible seizure focus already safely removed. I was privileged to have access to superb medical care and skilled physicians. I was blessed with loving friends and family who offered support.

At the same time, I was stubborn enough not to allow seizures, headaches, or unsteadiness alter my goal to be a pediatrician. I admired the strength of the forces that allowed me to leave the vortex of persistent illness, though I knew it would be a long time before I could live without fear of its return.

The summer of 2003 was a season of freedom. Like a molting bird, I gradually weaned off various medications until only what was necessary remained. As I gained strength, the headaches I'd experienced since surgery decreased in intensity and frequency. Eventually I stopped taking gabapentin, the medication that treated the post-operative headaches. As more and more days passed without seizures, I persuaded Dr. Rodgers to allow me to also discontinue one of my two anti-seizure medications. Roughly six months after surgery, I said goodbye to my long companion, carbamazepine, until only lamotrigine remained. I probably can't do justice in describing my feelings here, how wonderful I felt throwing away bottles of medication and loosening the ties that bound me to epilepsy.

When I discarded the medications, my constant attendants—worry and fear—slipped away, too. At first, like a crutch, I was afraid that reducing my meds, and pretty much anything else, might provoke a seizure. Epilepsy was like an evil queen that stalked children's fairy tales—retaliatory and powerful, refusing to be cast aside. But weeks, then months, passed without a moment of déjà vu, unusual twinge, or a seizure. With time, I believed that epilepsy had moved on without me.

24

THEN ONE DAY in mid-October everything changed again.

At the end of a particularly long day at the hospital, I was relieved to finally drive home to a quiet house and a warm bed. Since I hadn't had seizures for more than three months, the required period for a Wisconsin driver to operate a motor vehicle without restrictions, I was grateful to drive independently again. A kaleidoscope of fall colors splashed on the tree branches and the setting sun cast a brilliant orange shadow on the landscape. I hummed a familiar tune along with the radio and was content.

Suddenly and inexplicably, the music sounded as if it were at the end of a long tunnel. My hands tingled and involuntarily gripped the steering wheel just as an all-too-familiar heat ascended from my lower abdomen. I listened to the start of rhythmic swallowing and smacking lips as if I were an observer watching the eerie scene. The portion of my brain that held onto cogent thoughts screamed: *This can't be happening!*

Even in the absence of my right temporal lobe, the crescendo continued. In a last moment of luck and focus, I managed to pull my car safely out of traffic. When I rolled to a stop along the side of a residential street, I slumped back and relinquished control to the overpowering seizure.

My left foot pounded against the worn rug next to the brake pedal, controlled by some untamable electrical current that was stronger than my will to stop it. I knew I needed help. I tried to beckon a couple strolling down the quiet street with my remaining sliver of consciousness. Trapped both by the seizure and my increasingly warm car, I strained to roll down the window but fumbled unsuccessfully. Somewhere in the distance, I heard a repetitive high-pitched staccato yelping.

Was that me?

Minutes or hours later, the seizure was over. I rested my head against the steering wheel of my car and cried. My confusion floated away like dark clouds after a storm and permitted my mind to race down the path of possibilities of what a seizure so soon after surgery could mean. Did I have a post-operative bleed? Was there a cyst in my head that created excess intracranial pressure? Was this a sign of meningitis? Most of all I worried: did the seizure mean surgery didn't work?

Before I gave in to panic, I decided to page the neurosurgeon, Dr. Isaac, to get his opinion. With clumsy hands, I opened the previously impenetrable car door and tumbled onto the grassy curb. I crawled across the cool grass to a nearby tree and propped myself against the trunk to stay upright. I fumbled through my purse to retrieve my cell phone but the numbers were almost impossible to see in the fading light of the dusky sky above.

Slowly, I tried to dial the series of numbers that would contact Dr. Isaac. Despite my best efforts, my fingers were unruly lumps of dough that didn't respond well to my thoroughly clouded thoughts. The call I waited for never came. I rested my pounding head against the tree trunk and fought off beckoning sleep. Darkness fell and I leaned into the sturdy tree, confused, helpless, and alone.

Eventually, I summoned enough energy to study the confusing keypad of my phone again. This time I found the button that allowed me to call "Home."

Two long rings before there was a voice on the other line.

"Andrew?" I garbled.

"Kristin. You're crying. Are you okay?"

"I've had a seizure," I slurred. "I was driving when it started, but I pulled over and I'm okay. Please come and get me."

Concern and disappointment thickened Andrew's voice. "I'll be right there. Where are you?"

"I don't know. One of the side streets off of Park Street, I think. I'm leaning on a tree. I can see Meriter Hospital from here."

"Stay there. I'll find you. I'm leaving right now."

I leaned my head on the trunk of the tree where my surgical scar, still tender though five months old, hurt when rubbed against the rough wood. I let my eyes close and drifted quickly into the dead sleep that'd threatened ominously ever since I left my car. With Andrew on his way, I knew could rest.

Later, I roused and saw my husband running down a street lit by a last sliver of sunlight. His arms were wide open and tears streamed down his face. He jogged up to my tree and pulled me into his embrace. "I'm so sorry, are you OK?" he wept. "I'm so sorry, are you OK? I'm so sorry."

My tears of relief and mourning joined his. I was relieved to be safe but knew that my seizure pushed me across the chasm back into a life of precariousness and uncertainty. After a brief sojourn, epilepsy was back to stay.

* * *

E

One of the most frustrating consequences for many adults living with epilepsy is the inability to drive independently. The laws pertaining to drivers with epilepsy vary from state to state. The most common requirement for people with epilepsy is that they must be seizure-free for a specific period of time and submit a physician's evaluation of their ability to drive safely. In Wisconsin, a person with epilepsy may hold a valid driver's license if they've been free from seizures for three months.

Some states carry exceptions for those who can prove that they're medically stable. Patients who suffer seizures as a result of a medical condition that's been cured, whose seizures occur only when asleep, or who may be able to predict their seizures in order to ensure that they don't lose consciousness behind the wheel of a moving vehicle may be exempt from such restrictions or may have fewer restrictions.

25

WHEN I FINALLY got in touch with Dr. Isaac, he instructed me to go to the hospital for evaluation. Dr. Jones, the Emergency Department (ED) physician who'd been my supervising physician just a few nights before, met me in the ED. I enjoyed working with Dr. Jones and learned a lot from his vast knowledge of emergency medicine.

A nurse wheeled me past Dr. Jones's workstation after a CT scan of my head was complete. I was outfitted in another ill-fitting paper gown and cursed with another throbbing headache. Without looking my way, Dr. Jones told a nearby resident that he was going to discharge the "seizure in Room 10."

How quickly I transformed from a collaborating colleague to a symptom with a room number. I made a mental note to address all my patients by name instead of by medical problem and to look past each chief complaint to the human within.

Andrew and I returned home from the ED and slept fitfully while we digested the reality that my seizures were back. Night after night for weeks, I tossed and turned and tried to combat the exhaustion that penetrated as deep as my bones. I wondered why it took so long to recover from a simple seizure. I still took lamotrigine daily and my work schedule was atypically light, but I felt as if I were swimming in a sleepy sludge that tugged at my limbs and slowed my thinking.

Eventually, I realized that my normally regular period was two weeks late. I also had intermittent waves of nausea—especially in the mornings—which I erroneously attributed to my irregular residency schedule. When I finally put two and two together, I sprinted to the nearest pharmacy.

Pregnancy test in hand, I locked myself in our bathroom, sat on the toilet, and read the small-print instructions word for word. I might've had a medical degree, but I wasn't sure how to pee on the stick. I wanted to get it absolutely right. After I mustered up the confidence and did the deed, I placed the innocent white stick on the bathroom floor and waited the designated three minutes, an eternity.

Three minutes was longer than needed, however, because within seconds an acid-blue color whisked across the view bar and left a brilliant blue PLUS sign bright enough to make me squint. I pulled the stick closer to make sure and my heart raced. *This can't be!* I thought. *Can I really be pregnant?*

Addressing my disbelief, I fished in the box for the remaining test. I re-checked the instruction packet to make sure I was really doing it right, and re-tested myself. I eked out a few dribbles the second time, but enough to trigger the same reaction I'd witnessed minutes before. Light blue traversed the expectant white view bar, followed seconds later by the appearance of an unmistakable PLUS. I sank to the floor, clutching the two positive tests in my hands as if they were as precious as a baby itself. We were going to be parents.

I couldn't wait to tell Andrew this news. Although we're both meticulous planners by nature, we'd never had a frank conversation about when—or if—we should have kids. I'd stopped taking birth control months before, but we were so focused on our schooling and careers in medicine and business that up until that moment, adding a child to the mix seemed impossible. My pregnancy wasn't planned, but I was confident that the chance to nurture and mentor a child would give us perspective about the daily ambiguity of our marriage with epilepsy.

I walked tentatively into the living room and approached the couch where he was reading a magazine. Without a word, I grabbed Andrew's hand and tugged for him to come with me but offered no clues.

"What is it?" he asked. "Are you okay? Did you have a seizure?" Andrew repeated his default question any time I ever looked tired or acted withdrawn.

"No," I said through my growing smile. "I need to show you something."

Andrew let me lead him through the bedroom and into our bathroom, where I proudly pointed to the two positive test sticks resting on the counter, both with their bright blue PLUSes arranged on display. He cocked his head and looked at me quizzically. "What are these?" he asked. "And why does it smell like urine?"

I giggled with happiness and pointed to the opened box resting on the floor. The black lettering on the top of the package read:

EPT Pregnancy Test
Fast, accurate results in minutes!

Andrew studied my face to make sure I wasn't playing a trick on him. He must've seen the excitement and joy in my eyes because a smile started to travel across his lips as well. He wrapped me in an embrace and sighed deeply. I wasn't sure how to read his reaction so I pulled back and watched his expression, looking for an answer. "The timing is perfect. Thirty-one is a great age to become a father," he said simply.

I felt like I could fly.

*   *   *

E

Years ago, women with epilepsy were discouraged from becoming pregnant. Both seizures and seizure medications were associated with poorly-defined risks to the mother and the fetus. After decades of documentation and retrospective studies, however, researchers found that although women with epilepsy have twice the risk (4-6%) of having a baby with birth defects compared to that of the general population (2-3%), greater than 90% of babies born to women with epilepsy are completely unharmed.

The most common birth defects that occur in babies of women with epilepsy include cleft lip and palate and heart defects. Spina bifida, a congenital defect of the spinal cord, also occurs with increased incidence compared to the general population. Minor abnormalities of the face, fingers, and toes may also slightly alter the baby's appearance.

The actual cause for the increased risk of fetal malformations is undetermined. It's possible that the birth defects are genetically related to the cause of a woman's epilepsy. Or the birth defects may be secondary to the effects of the anti-epileptic drugs used to control seizures. Another possibility is that birth defects may occur because the baby has an increased genetic susceptibility to harmful effects of medications.

Even though the large majority of babies of epileptic mothers are born without visible birth defects, there is a 2-6% risk that infants of epileptic mothers will experience developmental delay. The risk of developmental delay is highest in infants of mothers with poorly controlled seizures or in those who were taking more than one anti-epileptic medication during pregnancy.

Finally, because pregnancy changes every woman's metabolism, pregnancy also changes a mother's level of anti-epileptic drugs. Although most pregnant women with epilepsy will see no change in their seizures, about one third will have more seizures when they're pregnant. If a woman continues to have seizures during pregnancy, seizures, especially grand mal, may harm the fetus, especially if they occur during the last month of pregnancy or during labor. Even once the baby is born, the epileptic mother continues to be at risk. Seizures are more likely to occur in epileptic women during the post-partum period due to the combination of stress, sleep deprivation, and fluctuating hormones.

26

THE REVELATION that I was pregnant put the relapse of seizures in a whole new light. The ebb and flow of hormones with my monthly cycles had influenced my seizures since my teenage years. It made sense that the hormones associated with pregnancy might have revived the remaining abnormal electrical pathways in my fickle brain. As my abdomen grew, my dose of anti-epileptic medications increased accordingly to keep up with my increasing metabolism. While I was able to maintain the image of a blossoming pregnant woman by day, once every few weeks my nights were interrupted by paroxysms of pulsing heat, smacking and swallowing, and tingling of my left arm and hand. My seizures were back without a doubt, but now I was focused on protecting the growing new life within me.

My twenty-week ultrasound was performed on February 11th, exactly one year after I was admitted to the V.A. Hospital for inpatient EEG monitoring. Even though the events of the previous year hadn't produced a cure, the ultrasound of a growing baby represented renewal and a progression of life beyond seizures.

The ultrasound technician lathered jelly on my abdomen and gently moved the transducer as I lay on yet another crisp white gurney in the ultrasound suite. Gradations of white, black, and grey projected on the screen above and I strained to see the first discernible image of the baby inside. Because I knew the risks my medications posed, I was anxious to see a full, intact upper lip, a heart without defects, and a fully formed spinal canal. I pulsed with expectation that this simple test could provide answers to the crucial questions that'd brewed over the past several months.

Is it a boy or a girl?

Is the baby healthy?

Are there any physical or developmental effects from my medications?

Although I knew the pictures would give us an idea about the physical well being of our baby, two critical questions remained:

Will there be any lasting effects on the fetus from my seizures during pregnancy?

Will our child have seizures?

The projected image on the screen above evolved into something resembling a human and quelled my racing thoughts. The swimming arms and legs, two of each, were mesmerizing. Fingers and toes fluttered and turned as our baby moved around the womb. The ultrasonographer took measurements of the baby's femur length, head circumference, and abdominal girth. I breathed a sigh of relief each time she seemed satisfied with the recorded values. Andrew and I stole a glance across my bulging belly, our nervous fingers locked in a sweaty embrace.

When the ultrasonographer turned her attention to the area between the baby's legs, another floating shaft of tissue confirmed our suspicions. It was a boy. We gazed at his face when they switched to the high-tech four-dimensional ultrasound and fell in love with the perfect image of our son. His eyes were closed and his brow was raised in a way that already looked inquisitive. His nose was broad at the base and flattened at the end like his father's. His intact lips caressed his right thumb while he soothed himself in utero. I was awestruck at the miracle of new life.

The ultrasonographer printed several images of the baby and I held them close to my heart for the next four and a half months. The high-risk obstetrician reviewed the images and joyfully informed us that we had a happy, healthy, and robust boy. So far the icy fingers of my epilepsy hadn't been able to grasp him. Through my tears and raging hormones, I thanked God for our unexpected blessing.

When the ultrasound was complete, Andrew and I joined the pediatric residents who congregated down the hall in the newborn nursery as shifts changed. I proudly held out the grainy image of our son and smiled when I pointed out the eyes, nose, and sucking thumb to anyone who would listen.

That night, Andrew and I lay with our hands on my softly gyrating belly, alive with the little boy inside, and decided to name our son Alexander Thompson. Alexander because I'd always dreamed of having a baby named Alexander and Thompson because it's Andrew's middle name. We figured a young man with a name like Alexander Thompson Seaborg could be a president, a businessman, an astronaut, a tradesman, or anything he wanted to be. Like the moon, nothing would be out of reach.

I drifted to sleep with visions of the boy-to-be dancing underneath my eyelids. I looked forward to the excitement that each new milestone of parenting would bring—a first smile, first steps, or first time driving a car. I prayed that the arrival of our son would lead to a life no longer ruled by seizures.

*   *   *

Perhaps foolishly, I never did any in-depth research to find out what sort of risks my babies would face because of my epilepsy. I focused on curing my seizures instead of learning to live with them, so up until the day of the positive pregnancy test, I didn't expect that epilepsy and motherhood would ever co-exist in my life. Armed with a computer, a medical library, and a cluster of rapidly dividing embryonic cells in my abdomen, I set out to understand everything I could about pregnancy and epilepsy.

As I sifted through a pile of papers and studies, facts and statistics, I was increasingly anxious but still felt the odds were in my favor. It wasn't until I glanced across the final page of an "Information

Pamphlet for Women with Epilepsy"[24] that I found a statistic that will haunt me forever:

Babies born to mothers with epilepsy have a 3% chance of developing epilepsy in their lifetime. Babies born in the general population have a 1% chance.

I guess this was a risk we were going to have to take.

27
2004

DURING MY SENIOR resident rotation in the Neonatal Intensive Care Unit (NICU), my job was to attend all high-risk deliveries and lead the team of pediatric residents during newborn resuscitations. Most of the time, this job was simple and rewarding. We scrambled into delivery rooms like a team of blue-clad superheroes and gathered medical supplies for every contingency like a well-honed pit crew. After we prepped for the imminent delivery, we often had a few moments to settle back to our appointed spots in the corner of the delivery room and wait.

Sometimes the nursing staff called us with plenty of time to spare before the baby arrived. In the late winter of my senior year, these were my favorite times. I witnessed countless deliveries where mothers grunted "I can't!" while expectant fathers cradled their heads and coaxed them through pain and the fear. Some delivery rooms were serene and peaceful, while others were filled with family yelling support and making jokes about the baby's size or a mother's strength. No matter the setting, I always fought tears of awe every time a baby emerged into the world from the fluid-soaked depths of its mother.

It was a privilege to witness the shocked look on a baby's face as she opened her eyes to meet the world. During our evaluation and resuscitation, I loved watching the baby respond to the sensations of touch, sound, and sight. I relished the sight of translucent skin transforming from blue to pink and the sound of each new cry that welcomed the ambient air and swept the fluid out of a newborn's lungs. I loved the new fathers, reduced to a puddle of tender surprise, who sidled up to the resuscitation table, peered over my shoulder, and watched, mesmerized by life's first moments. Each time I handed over a dry and bundled baby to speechless parents, I loved to say, "He's perfect!" while I surreptitiously patted my belly and wished for the same scene to play out in my life.

Unfortunately, not every delivery was picture-perfect. Most of the time, we knew if the baby had a birth defect or major medical problem before the time of delivery, thanks to the accuracy of prenatal ultrasounds. Still, there were a few surprises.

I was working one night when we were called to an emergent Cesarean section of a baby who had an unexpectedly trapped hand poking out of the cushioned confines of her mother's uterus. Somehow, through twists and contortions in the womb, the baby's arm became stuck over her head. During the initial phase of labor, her mother delivered the baby's hand but was unable to deliver the rest of the baby.

I jogged down the hall with the pediatric team, following the gurney that carried the laboring mother. A group of concerned obstetricians swarmed around her. We hurried to scrub our hands and fingernails and donned our surgical masks, hats, and booties before we fanned out to our respective positions in the operating room. I stood sideways next to the infant warmer; my pregnant belly interfered with my ability to fit easily in tight spaces. I wondered what to expect while I watched the obstetric team make a quick incision to free the baby.

Moments later, the pediatric intern swiftly placed the baby on the warmer and we began our assessment and resuscitation. I reflexively dried and stimulated the baby and my anxiety decreased when I noted that she was breathing and crying spontaneously with a vigorous heart rate. Three of her four limbs flexed and extended as expected, but the fourth, the right arm, lay limply at her side like an azure balloon.

I touched and lifted her arm with hesitation. Her fingers looked like five blue sausages attached to a ballooned arm. Her entire arm jiggled like electric-blue Jell-O when I gently laid it back on the table. Soon I sensed the presence of the new father over my left shoulder. Instead of pronouncing the baby perfect and healthy, I explained that we would have the pediatric orthopedic team assess the baby's hand and arms promptly.

Tears welled in the father's eyes. Over the cacophony of the noisy delivery room, I gently asked him what they planned to name the baby.

"Elizabeth," he uttered through tears. "Just look at her," he continued. "Her eyes are exactly like her mother's! She has a dimple on her chin like me! And look at that thick head of hair! She's going to be a beauty."

I nodded and relaxed, ashamed that I'd thought the baby's deformed arm and hand would be all a new father would see. Instead, he saw beyond her obvious imperfections and focused on the beauty elsewhere. I wished for a moment that we all could be as authentic and true as a new, proud parent. Whether there was a discolored, swollen limb hanging without purpose or rogue electrical currents coursing through a brain, there was beauty in everyone.

Even this baby.

Even me.

*   *   *

As the weeks passed leading up to the delivery of our baby, I felt as if my life were mimicking an epileptic seizure. Time and again, I whipped full-force from one role to another. I jumped from physician to patient to expectant mother in a manner similar to the involuntary forceful movements of my limbs when I experienced a seizure. When I collapsed into bed each evening, my persistent dull headache and general exhaustion was reminiscent of the familiar post-seizure lethargy that marked many of my days. The obstinate ambiguity of what to expect for the little boy growing inside mirrored the uncertainty over which days would bring a new epileptic seizure. I fought back fear of how seizures affected our baby and tried to ignore the nagging truth that although I diligently followed all the rules of pregnancy and avoided alcohol, caffeine (mostly), the cat litter and soft cheese, our baby was at markedly increased risk of a birth defect or injury. I felt convulsed and fragile, tacking between invisible but tangible boundaries.

And yet, reveling in my dreams and excitement for motherhood, I was charged with expectation and anticipation. No matter which role I played—doctor, patient, wife or mother—I understood that unpredictability was as important and necessary to life as breath. I acknowledged the unsettled and unknown as things to discover rather than fear. A new and strengthening inner peace chased away my demons.

After years of fighting, I accepted that epilepsy is beyond my control. Patient outcomes are to some degree beyond my control. Our baby's future was unpredictable but full of promise. Whatever I don't know is OK. My life is OK. I embraced the uncertainty and relished the surprises that came with each day.

Part III: The Mother
2004—2009

28

THE MORNING OUR SON was born began no differently than most summer days with the exception that sleep eluded me. The light brewed early on the banks of the horizon and spread quickly across the smoldering earth. The dew lining the grass turned to vapor that dissipated in the summer heat. I lumbered out of bed before my alarm clock, so ready to deliver our son.

It was one week and five days past my expected due date. I was finally scheduled for an induction to roust Alex from his comfortable spot in my womb. We'd already packed our bags—and loaded them into the car on three separate occasions thanks to false alarms—so there wasn't much to do except wait. My obstetrician instructed me to call the hospital at 8 A.M. to request a room number and bed assignment. That left me three endless hours before I could do anything. I sighed and heaved my swollen body toward the kitchen to make some tea. It was going to be a long day.

I showered and dressed in the maternity clothes that barely fit over my bulging body and walked the length of our condo to calm my nerves. I wanted to make sure everything was in order. In Alex's room, the crib sheet was pulled taut against a brand new mattress and his freshly washed blue baby clothes hung in the closet in chronological order. His diapers were arranged in perfect rows in the bureau, and there was a bouquet of diaper creams arranged on the side of the changing table. The light green walls of his room were stenciled with playful images of animals and an embroidered blanket hung carefully over the top of the rocking chair. I touched his clothes, toys, and books and smiled. I'd imagined our son in this room for so many months. Soon he would be home.

When I returned to the kitchen, I double-checked the fridge for the extra food I bought for Andrew to eat while I was in the hospital. I found milk, plenty of cold cuts, and a few treats we didn't normally buy, tucked away and waiting. The bills were paid, my hospital pager was disconnected, and my cell phone was charged so we could call friends and family with the good news. I was ready to get in the car and have a baby.

The microwave clock gleamed 6:13. There were still hours to wait.

Morning television filled the rest of the void until it was time to call the hospital at 8:00. The soft-voiced triage nurse issued a bed number and instructions to check in and we were finally ready.

Andrew and I spent most of the twenty-minute ride to the hospital in nervous silence. I couldn't help but compare our commute to a similar one fifteen months before, when my bags were packed not with baby clothes and diaper cream, but with warm pajamas and magazines to use while I recovered from surgery. When we crested a hill on our way downtown, I reflected on the crescendos and dips in our lives during the preceding eighteen months. I'd travelled from depression and despair in the months prior to surgery, confusion and weariness in the weeks to months afterwards, to elation and anticipation as our baby grew inside. The birth of our son would mark our transformation from a couple to a family. We knew our lives would be indelibly changed when the sun rose again tomorrow.

I announced my name at the main desk once we finally arrived at Meriter Hospital and we were given instructions to the room where Alex would be born. A cheerful nurse joined us and handed me a hospital robe. Her eyebrows rose in question when she reviewed my health history and noted "temporal lobectomy" and "epilepsy" listed in my problem list. She strapped a monitor onto my engorged abdomen when I settled back onto the bed. The reassuring rhythm of Alex's heartbeat was audible to everyone in the room. I caressed my active belly, vibrating with playful fetal kicks and bumps, and thanked God for the privilege to take part in one of the greatest miracles of all.

* * *

After a flurry of activity, Andrew and I rested quietly on the couch in the delivery room without much to do. The contractions began but were scarcely noticeable. Eventually, my labor progressed and the anesthesiologist placed an epidural. I settled back into my bed, numb and comfortable. We watched more daytime television than we'd ever seen, held hands, and waited.

Afternoon melted into evening and the contractions recorded on the monitor became more frequent and substantial. Alex continued to kick and tumble inside as if he knew that his world was about to change. Finally, the obstetrics resident came in and announced that I was fully dilated and it was time to push. I watched the buzzing beehive of medical personnel prepare for the delivery while still numb from the epidural and unaware of my pain. We were anxious to meet our son.

Forty-five minutes later, a squirming, red, juicy Alexander Thompson Seaborg entered the world. When the obstetrician handed him to me, I resisted the urge to examine the wriggling infant as I would any other newborn. Still, my curious hands stole a moment to study his body while the nurses cleansed and dried him. His perfect soft spot was exactly where it belonged. His spine was normal without any of the characteristic dimples or defects that come with spina bifida or any other myriad deformities that my medications could cause. His mouth opened symmetrically when he cried, his eyes squeezed tight to block out the shock of the outside world. His hands were clenched in perfect balls, his long, post-term fingernails stained dark from the muddy water from which he came. His toes splayed and curled in rhythm with his cries. I brought him to my chest to study his face. His dimpled nose sniffed and searched for a breast where he could suckle. He was perfect.

I spent the rest of the night suspended between exhaustion and elation. I ran my hands over our baby each time he fed and admired the cosmic work of art resting in my arms. Alex was a palpable reminder that life beyond seizures is real. He was a bundle of promise and a package of hope. I couldn't remember a time when I felt more alive.

29

IN MANY WAYS, motherhood came naturally to me. Alex was a needy baby, but in time we figured out the various ways to bump, jiggle, swaddle and sway him into baby oblivion. I lived in a haze of astonishment and humility during our first week at home. It was remarkable that a pint-sized creature could make me feel flush with pride and profoundly self-conscious at the same time.

In my sleep-deprived and overwhelmed state, I fluctuated between awe of his new life and humbled by my human inadequacies. I resolved to fight with all my resources to raise Alex outside of the shadow of epilepsy.

I will try my best to raise you with dignity, I whispered to Alex's curled ears, ruffling the remains of the fine dark hair left on his earlobe from birth.

I will do everything in my power to let you know that you are loved, I mumbled as I pressed a warm kiss into his wrinkled forehead.

I will love you no matter your physical and cognitive capabilities, I muttered into the creases of his hands as he curled his inchworm fingers around my lips.

I will fight with all my might to keep my epilepsy away from you, I murmured while I caressed his perfect, round head.

These promises made, time and again, always brought tears to my eyes. The hope in my heart fought the reality that Alex, too, could

be vulnerable to constantly threatening seizure activity. I knew that
the modern foreign chemicals designed to keep my seizures at bay
might've affected his cognitive potential. And yet he'd already survived
nine months of physical and developmental challenges and arrived
unscathed. Time and again, I held Alex close to my heart and hoped
that he might never walk burdened with the chains that bound me.

* * *

The week before Alex was born, I graduated from my pediatric
residency program at the University of Wisconsin. Eleven years of
relentless studying, grueling exams, and nights alone in the small
call room of the hospital paved the way to a coveted license to
practice pediatrics on my own. The arrival of our son made further
training in a pediatric subspecialty unappealing. Now that there
was a baby at home, I didn't want to spend any more nights away
working and therefore sought the predictable schedule of a primary
care pediatrician.

When I first looked for jobs in Madison—a city teeming with
college graduates, medical professionals, and more doctors per
square mile than anywhere else in the country—there were none to
be found. Eventually I accepted a position at a small private clinic
forty minutes away from home. During the nine months that I made
the commute to rural southern Wisconsin, I swore at the traffic and
cursed the crowded road that kept me away from my son. When I
was offered a position as an inpatient pediatrician, or hospitalist, at
the University of Wisconsin later that year, I jumped at the chance.

It felt like I was returning home when I settled back into the
familiar halls and routines at the U.W. Hospital eighteen months
after I left. Still, there were some notable and welcome differences.
My new long white coat was emblazoned with my name next to the
bright red University of Wisconsin crest. My previously omnipresent clipboard was replaced with a small pack of papers with dense
notes—the resident doctors and medical students recorded most
of the mundane data. Instead of fighting for position in a pack of

medical trainees trampling down the halls, I led the group, guided the discussions, and directed the care of our patients.

Through this, however, one thing that changed very little was my epilepsy. When my seizures came back five months after surgery, they planted themselves firmly in other, less accessible locations within my brain. Initially, as an attending hospitalist at U.W., my seizures were infrequent. They occurred almost exclusively at night, so I was able to keep epilepsy hidden from my colleagues, staff, and students. I worried every day that a seizure would occur during morning rounds or when I interacted with patients, but only those who were working at the same hospital two years previously had any knowledge of my medical history.

It was around this time that Dr. Rodgers and I embarked on a long, taxing, and still ongoing series of medication trials and failures. There were periods of success and improvement, but every anti-epileptic drug I tried eventually lost its battle.

Months wore on and epilepsy again gained strength. I learned to recognize the new warning signs, or aura, that a seizure may be coming. Prior to surgery, the sensation of déjà vu was a reliable sign that a seizure would follow. After my damaged hippocampus was removed, the déjà vu was gone. The new signs were the abrupt onset of nausea and dizziness combined with a flash frontal headache. When I felt this characteristic combination of symptoms, I looked for a corner or a chair where I would be safe and out of view in case a seizure took over.

Despite my fears, not all auras led to a seizure. When I weaned off one medication and moved on to the next, I experienced auras with an increasing frequency. Consequently, I was well-acquainted with a multitude of hidden hospital corners and secluded workspaces.

* * *

E

As I increasingly accepted epilepsy as a permanent fixture in my life, I found comfort in reading the literature as if I were trying to solve a giant cosmic puzzle. Though what I found invoked a deep sense of fear, I hoped that knowledge would somehow give me power to ward off the potentially detrimental effects of recurrent seizures.

While I read through the studies about cognitive decline, mood disorders, and stigmatization with trepidation, it wasn't until I learned more about Sudden Unexplained Death in Epilepsy (SUDEP) that I feared for my future.

The mortality rate for people with epilepsy is two to three times higher than would be expected in a healthy population. The risk of sudden death in epilepsy patients is 24-times higher than what is seen in the general population. SUDEP accounts for 7-17% of deaths among people with epilepsy.[25]

No one knows what causes SUDEP, but patients who are identified at greater risk are male, patients with brain lesions, developmental delay, a history of uncontrolled grand mal seizures, and patients who aren't compliant with their medications or whose dose of medication is too low. Patients with increased seizure frequency may be at greater risk for SUDEP, although even patients with as few as one seizure per year are at more danger of dying than the general population.

Though I found shadows of my history in many of the studies that predicted chronic seizures and poor outcome, I consoled myself with the knowledge that I was a successful physician, a wife, and mother. Still, I felt my fists clench in nervous anticipation as I read the bleak results of study after study. How long would it be before my house of cards crumbled?

30

LIFE EVENTUALLY FELL into a modestly predictable rhythm considering the accepted unknowns of living with epilepsy and parenting a toddler. Alex brought such joy and energy to our lives that it wasn't long before Andrew and I wanted to expand our family. Although we knew the risks epilepsy posed to my health and a baby's health, we hoped that with thoughtful planning and careful monitoring, a second child would be within our reach. Perhaps most importantly, we weren't willing to let the ugly reality of seizures alter our hopes and dreams. Therefore, when Alex was fifteen months old, we decided it was time to take another leap of faith and have a second child.

Since my pregnancy with Alex was a surprise, we were more thoughtful about our decision this time. I was on reasonable doses of two anti-epileptic medications, which placed a fetus at higher risk of congenital malformations. However, the risk of birth defects associated with my medications at the time, lamotrigine and levetiracetam, was relatively low compared to some of the other available anti-epileptic drugs. When I mentioned to Dr. Rodgers that I wanted to become pregnant, he recommended a high daily dose of folic acid to decrease the risk of congenital anomalies. I closely monitored my sleep and stress levels. Although I continued to experience auras of fleeting nausea and dizziness, by the time our second baby was conceived I hadn't had a seizure in three months.

But even careful preparation couldn't alter the electrical irritability of my brain. Mid-way through my first trimester, my complex partial seizures returned. During the sixth month of my pregnancy, I came home after a long day at the hospital feeling tired and edgy. The pediatric ward was full of sick children, and I'd worked until late in the evening the prior night while on call. Andrew was scheduled to work late, so I planned to feed Alex a quick, simple dinner before we both went to bed.

Alex smiled in his high chair and babbled to himself while I warmed up some Gerber ravioli and got him some milk and fruit. My abdomen jumped and jerked when the unborn baby stretched his limbs. I tried to ignore the repeated short auras that heralded the possibility of an oncoming seizure.

"Did you have a good day at Patti's?" I asked Alex. I feigned a smile and refused to acknowledge the challenging evening ahead.

"Good day!" Alex cheered through a mouthful of pasta. "We made dot dots!" He pointed to his bag and I pulled out a crumpled piece of construction paper adorned with random dots of bright paint. "I play with friends," he said proudly. At twenty-one months, Alex was a social child who played easily with other children. His ubiquitous smile disarmed even the most exhausted adults.

After dinner, I watched Alex play with his toys in the family room. He made the couch a pretend parking lot and *vroomed* his toy trucks along the leather cushions. I smiled in amusement, but each time I looked over to admire his handiwork, another aura washed over me.

The auras made me feel as if I were a light on a dimmer. It felt as though an unknown powerful source was repeatedly turning my aberrant electrical pathways from off to the dim setting. It was only a matter of time before my subconscious could no longer keep the unruly circuitry at bay. I knew I had no control over when I would progress 120 Watts into a seizure.

I thought briefly about calling Andrew and asking him to come home, but quickly decided against it. I must be overreacting. My weariness after a stressful day invariably exacerbated my fear of seizures.

After a short while, I washed Alex's face and changed him into his pajamas. I read to him while turned slightly sideways on the rocking chair, my growing abdomen resting on one knee so I could I heave Alex to the opposite side. I turned the pages of our well-loved version of *Goodnight Moon* and rested my head atop Alex's prickly blond hair. The warmth of his body coursed through me and quelled the fear the auras produced. Aura after aura after aura made for a disturbing backdrop to a quiet scene. I focused on the tactile pleasure of Alex's wet, coarse hair that caressed my cheek and the soft, toddler belly under my hand that moved with the ebb and flow of sleepy breaths. Could I make epilepsy go away if I just ignored it? Was this much love and contentment as powerful as the strongest anti-seizure medication?

I tucked Alex in to his crib and kissed him good night.

"Nigh-nigh, Mama," he called as I stepped softly out of the room.

"Good-night, my Love, good-night," I whispered and disappeared into the hall.

As soon as I returned to the family room to straighten the toys, the auras escalated until I sat down. I bent down to pick up a wayward truck when… blackness.

*   *   *

I awoke later with a throbbing, bitten tongue and sore, quivering muscles. My head was pounding and felt as heavy as a kettle-ball. I studied my surroundings and searched for clues to decipher what'd happened. My maternal semi-consciousness roused and I remembered that Alex lay sleeping in the other room. If I'd waited only a few moments longer before putting him to bed, my seizure could've unfolded in front of him. Should I teach my bright, perfect toddler how to call 9-1-1?

I roused my spent body off the floor and clutched my pregnant belly while I rubbed the emerging bump on my forehead where I must've hit the floor. I clumsily plucked the numbers on the phone that would reach Andrew at work before I melted back into the carpet.

* * *

Andrew called our next-door neighbors and the obstetrician's office as he sped home. I was still lying on the floor and slipping in and out of awareness when our neighbors, Brenda and Alice, let themselves in. Brenda immediately went to Alex's room to check on him while Alice helped me to the couch where I fell into a deep, dreamless sleep.

The obstetrician on call recommended that we go to the hospital for evaluation. Brenda and Alice stayed with Alex, and I walked into the ED leaning heavily on Andrew's arm. A familiar nurse met us at the entrance. The look in her eyes shifted from one of recognition to confusion when she studied my tentative gait, heavy eyelids and swollen abdomen.

"You've had a seizure?" she asked, the tone of her voice ticked up a notch. "Then we need you in a wheelchair," she declared. I was back in patient mode: yesterday I was the one giving orders, today it was my turn to be ordered around.

I was wheeled into one of the rooms with a view of the central workstation that vibrated like a busy train depot. Nurses and staff moved in and through the central area as doctors paused to consult each other and document on one of the computers in between seeing patients. I moved to a bed and the nurses checked my vital signs, verified my medications, and took a brief history.

In between questions and periods of sleepiness, I noticed two of my colleagues conversing outside the windowed doors of the exam room. One of the men, a pediatric resident who'd worked with me the previous month, turned his head to survey the emergency department and his eyes caught mine. Caught off-guard, he looked quickly at the white board that displayed the chief complaint of each patient. When he read "seizure" in my designated slot, he glanced back into my small room and tried his best to appear unfazed. "Are you okay?" he mouthed while simultaneously gesturing to my bed and the white board ahead.

I mustered a feeble smile, nodded convincingly, and hoped he wouldn't detect the shame I felt every time my epilepsy was exposed or my embarrassment that I was lying defenseless in a gurney behind glass doors.

Dr. Resident busied himself with the charts in front of him and looked relieved that he wouldn't have to participate in an awkward conversation. He quietly moved on to a different patient in a room down the hall.

The obstetrician on call stopped by and reviewed the data from the fetal monitors. The kindly Emergency Department physician (whom I also considered a colleague) spoke through his brillo-brush mustache with puffed pillows of air in a soft, reassuring tone when he gently moved my disheveled hair to check the growing bump on my forehead. Finally, the doctors declared that my unborn baby and I had endured the grand mal seizure unscathed. We received the news with tremendous relief, especially since we knew that generalized seizures in the third trimester of pregnancy pose higher risk of fetal injury and distress. I was discharged with instructions to rest at home for one or two days while my body and the baby recovered.

Early the following morning, I called a colleague and asked her to cover my patients at the hospital while I rested and recovered from the seizure. I waited nervously when her phone rang repeatedly. I tentatively explained my request when she finally answered.

"I had a grand mal seizure last night," I explained, "and was in the ED for a while. I feel terrible and the obstetrician gave me instructions to stay home today. Would you be able to look after my patients today?"

My colleague gave a long sigh that built like a tsunami while she contemplated my request. "I guess I can help," she muttered begrudgingly. "I have a really busy day today, too."

"I know, and I'm sorry." My pleading tone revealed how much I loathed asking favors of others. "I wouldn't be very good at my job today." Although we were in the profession of taking care of others' ailments, illness in a physician is considered a sign of weakness.

She cut me off. "That's fine. I've got it."

"Thank you."

"Oh, and I hope you feel better." She threw out the last statement as an afterthought and hung up abruptly.

I fell back into my bed and lay flat as if the weight of the world was pressing on me. I hated feeling like I was shirking work because of epilepsy. I hated hiding my illness, and worse, having it exposed. I hated my shame of something that was a part of me but not because of me—something that I likely would never be able to control. Fatigue and frustration overwhelmed my aching body and ushered in a long, deep sleep.

31

THE CHAIR OF the Department of Pediatrics was known affectionately to some as the "Ice King." Dr. Cohen wore fitted grey suits
that perfectly matched his flawless helmet of grey hair and his trim
salmon lips. It was easy to hear him traversing the clean white halls
of the Children's Hospital each morning, his dress shoes clicking
with purpose against the linoleum floor. He ran a tight ship, kept the
medical students and residents on their toes with countless questions,
and had high expectations of every member of his staff and faculty.

Although I believed my experiences as a patient made me a better
physician, I knew my boss would think otherwise. With this in mind,
I hid behind a wall of feigned energy and vigor, even though it took
several days before my muscle pain and recurrent auras resolved
after my grand mal seizure. In a similar manner, I ignored the fact
that the increasing doses of anti-epileptic drugs required during
pregnancy frequently left me fatigued and nauseous.

Several days after my grand mal seizure, Dr. Cohen requested a
meeting. He was already seated at the faux wood table in the center
of his office when I arrived. With a tight smile, he invited me to
sit. I waited while he meticulously opened a single-serving packet
of Crystal Lite tea and poured it precisely into a waiting water jar
without spilling a single granule of aspartame-laden sweetener. He

stirred his drink and shook the bottle vigorously until the water transformed to an unnaturally pink elixir. Once his ritual was complete, Dr. Cohen raised his grey eyes to meet mine.

"I hear you asked Dr. Knight to work for you last Friday," he announced.

I knew this would come up. A thousand explanations and excuses sprang to my mind while Dr. Cohen calmly sipped his tea. Eventually I decided to explain with the best excuse I had: the truth.

"I was diagnosed with epilepsy at age eighteen," I began. The color rose in my cheeks as it always did when I talked about my seizures. "I've tried multiple medications and had surgery to remove the focus of my seizures two years ago," I paused to study Dr. Cohen. His expression was unchanged but his drink was held still mid-arc to his mouth. "For the most part, I do pretty well with my current medications and I rely on a predictable aura that warns if any small seizures are coming. When I'm pregnant, my hormones lower my seizure threshold and put me at risk for more frequent events."

Dr. Cohen lowered the luminescent pink drink.

I swallowed nervously and continued, "Last Thursday night I had a grand mal seizure, probably related to my hormones and fatigue. I stayed home Friday to recover." My last word hung in the air and I waited to see how my supervisor would react.

"Oh…my," he said as a cloud crossed his slate-grey eyes. "When was the last time this happened?"

Mind scrambling, I knew I needed to answer very carefully so as not to imperil my standing in the department. I wondered whether I should try to appeal to his sympathetic side and tell him the whole story from beginning to end, or whether I should downplay everything I'd been through and just tell him that I'd work as hard as ever to achieve department goals.

In the end, I took the middle road. We talked about the latest grand mal seizure and I attributed it to the hormones of pregnancy. I didn't tell him about the seizure I'd had one month before or the one that followed a few weeks after that. I also didn't share that the constant expectations to see more patients, teach students and residents, and spearhead the implementation of a new electronic medical record were contributing to my stress and sleep deprivation and therefore probably contributing to my loss of seizure control.

In retrospect, the content of that conversation was one of the final building blocks of the wall that divided my existence into two separate parts: Kristin with Epilepsy and the Kristin that the Rest of the World Saw.

When the meeting ended, Dr. Cohen sloshed the remaining dregs of his drink around the bottom of the bottle contemplatively and spoke. "I'm glad you told me about what happened last week." I was hopeful that empathy would accompany his understanding. Instead, his overcast eyes locked with mine and he declared, "I'm sure you know this can't ever happen again."

Despite what I revealed or withheld, from that moment on I believe I became to him the Woman With Epilepsy. Men and women with lesser qualifications received promotions and recognitions while I remained in a year-to-year position. In quiet moments, I wondered privately if Dr. Cohen's response and intolerance for my absence from work would've been the same if I'd shared instead that I had diabetes, cancer, asthma, or any of the other frustrating chronic illnesses that weren't accompanied by stigma. With effort, I ignored the cynical inner voice that told me that epilepsy is an unacceptable unknown for a physician. I worked hard, worked well with my colleagues, and had a talent for putting children at ease.

But my seizures were what mattered most.

*   *   *

Three weeks remained before my due date. At times, I welcomed being at work, which kept my mind off the baby and gave me time away from our adorable yet very active toddler at home. On a cool September day, I sat in my long, skinny office and looked out the tiny window at the impenetrable brick wall of the building next door. Hardly an executive view, but a window nonetheless. I put my feet up on my desk and took a moment to appreciate the robust fall breeze and the rustling crinkle of falling leaves dancing against the glass.

I closed my eyes and dreamt of what our second son would look like. Would his eyes be green like Alex's or brown like mine? Would he have Andrew's uncanny ability to fill any silence with words or would he be more introverted? After only a few quiet moments, my pager rang. I wearily raised the small device to read the text. "Call Dr. Volt about an admission."

It would be a long afternoon.

Dr. Volt sent me a sixteen-year-old female who presented with fainting spells and anemia. I wrote preliminary orders and talked to the nurses on the pediatric ward before I looked up to see the patient, Amy, saunter down the hall accompanied by her father and her sister. Amy shuffled along with her dark eyes cast down and her expression empty, flanked by protective family members on both sides.

The nurses showed Amy to her room and passed me the clinic notes from Dr. Volt's office. I shuddered when I read through the file and noted several symptoms that would be alarming in any child: fainting with activity, severe anemia with a hemoglobin of 6.0, and an unintentional weight loss of ten pounds over the past two months.

I was nervous about what I would find when it was time to meet Amy; the clinic notes painted a picture of serious illness. So I was surprised to greet a smiling, wide-eyed teenager with arms sheathed in colorful tattoos. Her nose, eyebrow, upper lip, ear cartilage, and ear lobes were home to multiple silver studs. When she talked, I saw the platinum bar rooted in the middle of her tongue that forced her to talk with a slight lisp. She sat up in bed and laughed at a gossip magazine with her similarly aged sister. I observed Amy from the doorway and bit by bit found physical clues that were signs of her acute illness.

Amy's olive skin was darker than mine, but several shades lighter than her sister's, a sure sign of her profound anemia. Her chocolate eyes were ringed with thick, charcoal circles. Her fingernail beds were milky white, a testament to the paucity of red blood cells in her body. Her lips were pale and her face had the sallow, mustard hue of chronic illness.

"Hi Amy, I'm Dr. Seaborg," I said. "How are you doing today?"

"I'm great, thanks." Amy tried to maintain an upbeat demeanor even when she clearly felt otherwise. "How are you?"

"I'm fine," I said quickly. "I've read Dr. Volt's notes, but I was hoping you could tell me in your own words about the events that brought you to her office today."

I'd learned that when possible, it's best to get a medical history directly from each patient. Even with our best efforts, multitasking physicians can get some historical details wrong. From the perspective of a patient, I felt validated when a physician spoke to me as if I was sharing important information each time I recounted my story.

Amy glanced at her father and her sister and then began a narrative of what led to her hospitalization.

"I work at the Pizzeria Uno's on the West side," she said. "I've been working a shift three or four evenings after school and once each weekend for a while to save money for college.

"Yesterday, I lifted a heavy tray and suddenly felt weak. My vision changed and if felt like the room was spinning. As soon as I sat down and put my head in my hands, the feeling passed.

"Later yesterday afternoon, I lifted another heavy tray and my legs lost their strength. The room spun again, and I had tunnel vision. I think I fainted, but I'm not really sure. No one was with me then.

"When I told my father what happened, he took me to the doctor."

Simple enough, I thought. A teenage girl, who probably didn't have the time or interest to eat enough, felt faint when working waitress shifts in addition to a busy high school schedule. She looked a little pale, but there was nothing that couldn't be fixed with a quick blood transfusion and a lecture about the importance of eating well and getting plenty of rest.

I explained my plan to draw a few additional blood tests and arranged for a transfusion to treat Amy's anemia. I walked out of her room confident that I'd have the admission tied up before the on-call hospitalist came at 5:00 P.M.

But my quick assumptions made me avoid consideration of the true reason for Amy's anemia. Although it's common for menstruating girls to have mild anemia, the paucity of red blood cells in Amy's blood work almost certainly pointed to a more sinister problem. When the lab values trickled back in, I knew that I'd been fooled by Amy's cheerful facade, and my presumptive conclusions. The laboratory technician found an army of abnormally shaped and minimally functional white blood cells in Amy's blood—a characteristic sign of acute lymphoblastic leukemia.

I walked to Amy's room to tell her she would be transferred to the University Hospital for further evaluation and thought about my initial interview with her. Just beyond the reach of my conscious knowledge or intent, I carried multiple biases into her room. My biases unwittingly shaped and altered my beliefs about her illness and about Amy as a patient.

Did the fact that she was a teenage girl make Amy's symptoms or complaints less credible than an adult or a young child? Did the presence of her giggling sister make her anemia less significant or her pallor less grave? Did her tattoos and piercings make her more likely to make lifestyle choices that could lead to illness?

I knew the answer to these questions was an emphatic *No*, but I wondered how stereotypes or misperceptions unintentionally affected my clinical judgment. When I was the one in a gurney, did the fact that I was a pregnant woman alter the provider's opinions about the truth of my seizures? Did my multiple medication trials and failures mean to some that since there was no way to cure me now, there would be no way to cure me, ever? Did the fact that I have epilepsy lead others to believe that I'd never be a good parent, good wife, or good doctor?

I quietly scolded myself for succumbing to unfounded ideas, tastes, and opinions that altered how I thought about Amy. Her diagnosis was readily evident in her lab work, but others wouldn't be as easy. Now that I was finally entrusted to care for patients on my own, I promised to treat each child exactly as I would want to be treated. The walls created by years of preconceived notions and unfounded beliefs would take effort to dismantle.

32
2006

THE SCHEDULED INDUCTION of the delivery of our second son was exactly on his due date. My second pregnancy had been a bumpy ride of escalating medication doses, increasing seizure frequency, and several unplanned trips to the hospital. My obstetrician advocated for induction, hoping to avoid further complications. It was time to move on.

The evening before William's scheduled birth was a cool, fall night. The wind blew strong gusts that sent the abandoned leaves galloping across our concrete driveway to accumulate in a pile in a ditch beyond. Inside, our house was warm, alive and festive. One of Andrew's high school friends was in town for the night and we invited him and his spouse over for an impromptu dinner.

When I slipped out to grab the mail, I peered into the windows filled with light and admired my smiling husband and our gregarious two-year-old. Alex sat on his dad's lap and chatted animatedly with our visitors. The heartwarming scene inside the house energized me momentarily, but I knew I wasn't myself.

I'd pushed myself to the limit that week. My globe-like belly made it almost impossible to sleep and I was working long hours in effort to tie things up at work before maternity leave. I knew that seizures would find me soon.

When I returned inside, Andrew's friend, Mike, smiled at me from across the table. "So, tomorrow's the big day, huh?"

"Yes," I sighed. "And I'm ready to be done."

Mike took a generous bite of his pizza and a drop of amber-colored grease travelled onto his hand and down his forearm. "Have you had an easy pregnancy?" he pressed.

I glanced quickly at Andrew before I answered. "Yes," I lied. "The end is always difficult when you're so large and tired, but things have have gone pretty smoothly."

Mike and his wife were hoping to start a family. I didn't want to frighten them with the details of our unplanned trips to the Emergency Department and extra doctor's appointments because of epilepsy. We also had an unspoken rule to never dwell on the obstacles we met because of seizures. Alex was over two and never saw or heard of a seizure despite their fairly regular appearance. We didn't want to worry my parents and Andrew's parents so they had limited knowledge of the persistence of my seizures. Even Andrew had little idea about the escalating frequency of my seizures or my daily battle with the worry and trepidation that came with the ritual of monitoring my sleep, re-evaluating every unusual body sensation, and in locating safe corners to disappear in case a seizure suddenly developed.

After Mike and his wife left, Andrew and I cleaned the kitchen and packed our bags for the hospital. I was thrilled that it was almost—finally—time to meet William. I took the chance to appreciate the beautiful evening for a last time when I took a bag of garbage to the end of the driveway. Alex was in bed, our company was gone, and everything was set for our new baby's arrival.

I walked and listened to the familiar music of the leaves and the trees when an aura swiftly materialized. *I told you so,* Epilepsy seemed to taunt through the pulsing heat and confusion, *you can't deny that I'm a part of you.*

I saw Andrew at the other end of the driveway and walked to him slowly through the developing seizure. Later, Andrew told me that I walked to him with a blank stare and stood quietly before I abruptly became rigid. My unconscious body slumped into his arms and he carefully lowered me to the ground just as the jarring muscle contractions of the seizure began.

Andrew dragged my pregnant, convulsing body into the safety of our garage with effort. He placed my bobbing head on a pillow of recycled newspapers before he ran into the house to call 9-1-1.

* * *

A stranger's face hovered over me as the fog cleared.

I was lying on the cold, hard floor of our garage surrounded by unfamiliar lights and sounds. Off in the distance somewhere, someone was calling my name.

"Kristin? Kristin? Can you open your eyes for me?"

I managed a one-eyed glance at the concerned faces around me using all the strength I could muster. Just beyond the swell of my abdomen, I saw the furrowed brow of Andrew, who was leaning down to rearrange a blanket draped over my legs.

Where was I?

The unfamiliar man with a soft voice and a warm hand on my wrist introduced himself. "Kristin, my name is Dan. I'm from the Middleton EMS. Your husband called us tonight because you had a grand mal seizure that lasted about six minutes. We found you here on the floor of your garage when we arrived, and you're starting to wake up now. We're going to get you on to this gurney and head into the hospital to check on you and your baby."

Baby? Confusion blurred to panic when I remembered my scheduled induction the following day. Tears welled, and strong hands lifted my wayward body off the cold floor and onto a cool bed. I was rolled into the back of the ambulance where the air was warmer and the lights were brighter. Moments later, the familiar silhouette of my brother appeared at the ambulance's open back door. Jon's face flashed red and white with the blinking emergency lights. He nodded his hello and reassurance before he went into the house to keep Alex company. Andrew's lips brushed my cheek, the bed was secured, and the truck rolled away.

Once we were on the road, I felt a prick for the IV poke, a squeeze on my upper arm for the blood pressure measurement, and then the joyous return of gentle kicking low in my abdomen. I drifted back out of consciousness as the ambulance bumped down the roads of Madison to Meriter Hospital.

The tests done on the baby at the hospital confirmed that he wasn't in distress. I was admitted to the hospital for observation and Andrew went home to await the arrival of my parents, who were coming to stay with Alex the following morning. I spent the night alone in an outdated and sparsely used section of the obstetrics ward. My bed was lined with cushion-covered metal rails designed to protect me from injury in case I seized again. The door to my room was kept open with a straight view to the main desk where the nurses could watch me. When I got up to use the bathroom, a nurse quickly jumped up and held my forearm as I pushed my IV pole across the room.

Morning came with its usual promise of a clean slate. I travelled from the dingy ante-partum room to the official labor and delivery floor. Andrew arrived shortly after the fluid in my IV bag was switched from saline to Pitocin. We collapsed into each other's arms.

"I was really scared," he breathed. "I don't think it's recommended to have a huge seizure when you're forty weeks pregnant."

"You did exactly the right thing," I reassured him. "You kept us safe. William will be okay."

"How do you feel?" Andrew asked.

"Sore. My thoughts are a little cloudy. But the baby looks great on the fetal monitors, and I'm sure he's alright."

Andrew's eyes searched my face as if they were looking for the clue to feel confidant and calm too. Though I hated dealing with the after-effects of each seizure, I had empathy for those who watched when an untamed force recklessly overpowered my body.

William Kristofer Seaborg was born later that day, at 8:44 P.M., just an hour after the harvest moon dropped below a golden horizon. He was proportioned exactly the same as his older brother born twenty-seven months earlier: 8 lbs. 4 oz. and 20.5 inches long. His bald head was adorned with a thin layer of hair as fine and blond as the feathers that coat a new baby chick. His large eyes sparkled with hints of the bright blue that would remain. We were in love.

33

"BIG BRODDER" ALEX strode into the hospital the following day with his head held high and grandparents in tow. His matter-of-fact reaction to seeing his brother for the first time was, "Oh. That's baby Will."

Alex paused and examined the baby closely, like a tiger inspecting his prey. Tenuously, he asked, "Can I touch him?"

A series of magical, delicate interactions ensued. We were careful to keep Alex involved with Will from the very beginning. He participated in soothing the baby by rubbing him gently on the cheek or forehead. At home, Alex always knew where to find Will's favorite musical toy and a pile of burp rags.

To my delight, Alex found his own ways to adjust to the new addition. The first time I nursed Will at home, Alex ran to his room in a flurry. Seconds later, he came out carrying a two-inch plastic Fischer Price baby doll with his chest puffed out and standing at least an inch taller. Alex marched up to me, tall and proud, and held his toy out for inspection.

"This my baby Will," he announced. He then crawled up next to me on the couch, lifted his shirt, and "nursed" his baby, too. One infant suckled and one toddler chatted while my heart swelled with pride.

I've heard others say that the hardest part about having a new-born is the older toddler at home. As expected, Alex showed more flashes of temper and regressed to waking up at night again after his brother was born. He even asked us to take the baby back to wherever he came from. And although I was often tired and over-whelmed, I learned quickly that I was able to love two little boys as much as I loved one and that my lap was big enough to cradle both tightly and closely.

*　*　*

Towards the end of my pregnancy with Will, my neurologist pre-scribed a new medication in attempt to quell my persistent seizures. Zonisamide, or zonegran, was a relatively new medication in the United States though it'd been used in Japan for years. Afraid to expose my unborn baby to additional new toxins, I put off adding that medication to my daily regimen until after Will was born. I was ready to give it a try after the baby arrived.

I googled "zonisamide" while at home one night with a squirm-ing Will snuggling into my right shoulder. PubMed Health, the first website I visited, listed the warnings and advisories in a list that spanned three pages. I read the list meticulously and tried to prepare for what to expect. In bold letters, the text warned of possible nausea, vomiting, weight loss, changes in taste, diarrhea, constipation, heartburn, dry mouth, headache, dizziness, confusion, irritability, difficulty sleeping, difficulty with memory, tingling in hands and feet, uncontrollable eye movements, double vision, rash, peeling skin, back pain, stomach pain, pain with urinating, sores in mouth, easy bruising, difficulty speaking, difficulty walking, poor coordination, severe weakness, severe muscle pain, extreme tired-ness, loss of appetite, irregular heartbeat, and loss of consciousness.

Was that all?

The side-effect profile of zonisamide was enough to make me want to give up and stay with what I knew, however ineffective. A sense of melancholy crept over me as I sat, numb, in front of my computer. Before too long, I thought of my family, and my desire to free myself of seizures forever. I was no longer fighting a battle just for myself, but also for the two innocent little boys who depended on me for comfort and security. No matter the risks, I had to try.

Will squirmed from his slumber and nestled further into the crook of my neck. His rhythmic breathing pulled me back to the present. I closed my laptop and prepared to do the laundry, dishes, and bathe the boys. I remembered that success with anything—including the wriggling ball of baby boy resting next to me—takes a little bit of gumption and a lot of faith.

At the sink the next morning, I studied the two unfamiliar red and white lined capsules in the palm of my hand and hoped they'd be the magic potion that cured me. I whispered a silent prayer and swallowed them down.

The addition of zonisamide came with familiar but bearable exhaustion but thankfully, there weren't any life or limb-threatening emergencies. I welcomed one notable side effect: a decrease in appetite that led to a fifteen-pound weight loss over the next several months. Even though I took high daily doses of the new medicine, it wasn't long before the seizures returned.

First the nighttime episodes came back. In the middle of the night, I woke with repetitive swallowing and tingling in my left hand followed by a bite mark on my tongue the following day. Soon, I experienced identical episodes during the daytime hours with increasing frequency. Friends and family told me that I looked great with the weight loss and renewed energy after I adjusted to the meds. Desperate to have my health follow the picture-perfect mold of our early family life, I said nothing to anyone that the new fix wasn't entirely working. Instead, I dressed in my new, smaller clothes each morning and headed off to work after I kissed our darling boys goodbye. Privately, I wondered just how long my secret would be safe.

34

DESPITE MY BEST EFFORTS, I struggled to find work-life balance with two small children, a demanding job, and persistent seizures. I decided it was time to take a new path and switched jobs around Will's first birthday. I left my position as a hospitalist and accepted a job as a primary care pediatrician with a group that had an excellent reputation for being family-friendly with predictable work hours. With regular hours and a half-day off each week, I hoped for a better quality of life. I also looked forward to fewer stressful days since I would care for well children instead of the sickest ones at the hospital.

I was right about some aspects of working in primary care. The hours were regular, the administration considerate of the needs of working parents, and the children I cared for weren't acutely ill. However, my days in clinic were no easier than the days spent on the hospital floor. I hustled from exam room to exam room just as quickly as I'd sped down long hospital corridors in the past. My new patient population challenged me with a whole new set of illnesses: depression, anxiety, attention deficit disorders, parents who didn't love them, classmates who bullied them, and a lack of self-esteem and self-respect. I cared for a multitude of patients who were burdened with unplanned pregnancies, abusive families, substance abuse or gangs. I didn't have medicine to fix broken relationships or lack of self-worth. I was in over my head.

Contrary to most working parents, Monday mornings were my favorite part of the work week. Alex and Will left with Andrew for daycare at eight and I had a few extra hours in the house before my clinic started at eleven. The quiet house was most inviting after a weekend of running, squealing children who ran and jumped higher and further than a pack of kangaroos.

On a promising spring morning after a quiet coffee at the sunlit kitchen table, I was anxious to get the laundry done before I left for work. I opened the overhead dryer door quickly to move the wet clothes into the dryer. I stood with a pack of soggy clothes held against my chest and slammed my upper lip into the sinister door.

WHAM! The flash of pain was a reminder of the defect in my vision that remained after epilepsy surgery. Everything in the left upper quadrant of my visual field was permanently invisible because of the path the neurosurgeon took to reach the offending part of my brain.

"GOD!" I exclaimed. Tears sprang to my eyes.

Where was He anyway? The taste of blood filled my mouth. I grabbed my lip and sank to the floor in despair. "I'm tired of pretending that everything's OK," I cried. "I'm tired of running all the time, meeting other people's needs and feigning an image of order and control. I'm surrounded by chaos and I'm definitely not in control."

I sat on the cold tile floor and sobbed. No matter how many rules I followed, no matter how precisely I lived, I would never know what to expect. Whether in the form of a seizure, a medication side effect, or a swinging metal force outside of my field of vision, the reality of epilepsy always brought me to ground level.

I grabbed a towel, dabbed at my bleeding lip and went to collect my things at a glacial pace. I had a busy day at the office. I needed to keep moving and had no time for self-pity, wallowing, or wishing I were someone or somewhere else. My lip would stop bleeding, and epilepsy would not rule this day or any other day.

Epilepsy would not rule my life.

I went to the bathroom to examine my injury and re-touch my makeup before I left. My lip was swollen but the redness was easily disguised by lipstick. I smiled at myself in the mirror and pretended to introduce myself. No one would know. I purposefully collected my coat, purse, and shoes, and tucked my fearful, anxious, and defenseless self away into the unreachable caverns inside. With a last comb of my hair and dab of make-up, I transformed into the professional and mother known to the outside world.

35

THE SAME DAY I went to work with a swollen upper lip, I met two fifteen-year-old girls who were outwardly very similar but had important hidden differences. The first teen, Jennifer, was a sophomore in high school and one of four children from an affluent family. She lived most of her early childhood wanting for nothing, acclimated to luxury and accepting nothing less than perfection. Jennifer was fantastically aware of each faltering pang of discomfort and fleeting deviation from normal within her body. I saw Jennifer often for evaluation of stomach aches, indigestion, menstrual cramps, leg cramps, sinus pressure, dizziness, and fatigue. Numerous lab tests, physical exams and subspecialty referrals all came back negative.

I became Jennifer's pediatrician on her thirteenth birthday. During every office visit, Jennifer sat in a corner of the exam room and looked uninterested while her mother did most of the talking. Whenever I asked Jennifer directly about her symptoms, she mustered a sour face, clutched her side, and became animated with illness.

Then one day, an accident. Jennifer tripped over a kitchen chair and hit the side of her head. She didn't lose consciousness, she didn't feel nauseous, and she didn't become confused or sleepy. Three days after the incident, however, she noticed that her memory of a sporting event that'd taken place two days prior to hitting her head was a bit fuzzy. Jennifer and her mother became concerned about her memory in the context of the fall and she was seen in the local hospital Emergency Department. A CT scan of her head was normal and Jennifer was diagnosed with a mild concussion before she was discharged home. Even though Jennifer didn't have headaches previously, after her ED visit, she was crippled by them.

I saw Jennifer in the office several days later to follow-up on her headache and concussion. She laughed, smiled, and joked with the office staff as they prepped her for her visit. Still, when I walked into the room moments later, her mother exclaimed, "Just look at her! I don't think she's well. She says her head hurts very badly. Don't you think she should continue to stay home from school?"

After I did an exam, I smiled and tried to reassure Jennifer and her mother. I encouraged her to return slowly to activity, and suggested she take short walks as a first step to recovery. Both mother and daughter sighed and stood to leave. I had no doubt that they'd returning soon, with a new ailment.

Later that day, I saw Tiffany, also fifteen but who lived life on a different path. Tiffany was born with a congenital anomaly that made it impossible to straighten her neck and with a spine that rested painfully in a contorted "S" shape. Tiffany was unwilling to let her physical differences affect her goals in life. Beginning at a young age, her parents encouraged her to row canoes to strengthen her core muscles. As a teen, Tiffany was captain of a competitive crew team and worked as a waitress part-time. She intended to become a doctor one day.

Tiffany complained of severe headaches and neck pain. When I studied her profile, I noted that her neck was fixed with her head permanently tilted to the right. "I have to move my whole body to see the white board at school," she explained, "and I get sore by the end of the day."

"What do you do for the pain?" I asked.

"Well, sometimes I rest," Tiffany said as she readjusted her body to look at me, "and sometimes I take Tylenol. Physical therapy and massage help a little, too. Most of the time, I keep going because I don't have time to do anything else."

I washed my hands to do a physical exam and admired Tiffany's remarkable ability to deal with chronic discomfort at such a young age. When I felt along the side of her neck—an area that should be firm yet easily pliable underneath my fingertips—I felt a tight cord of thickly contracted muscle, evidence of her persistent pain.

"Whoa," I said, walking my fingers along the tight muscle. "Does this hurt?"

"No more than usual," she answered.

I arranged for more physical therapy visits as well as follow-up with orthopedic and rehabilitation medicine specialists. She refused my offer for additional medications for pain. Final exams and a crew event were coming in the following weeks, and she didn't want anything to jeopardize her performance.

I thought of my own children after my encounters with Tiffany and Jennifer. When faced with a challenge, I hoped to teach them to be more like Tiffany, who stared down adversity, and less like Jennifer, who leaned into it. Something important was lost in their generation of helicopter parents and coddled children—the resilience to tackle a problem with inner strength instead of relying on others to make it better. If I could teach our kids to cultivate resilience, we could give them both roots *and* wings to encourage them to one day fly on their own.

I struggled with resilience versus complacence through my experiences with seizures and illness. If I could remain strong, I would have every opportunity to make my own choices and choose my own path.

Like Tiffany, I wanted to choose resilience every time.

*   *   *

It's been postulated that patients with epilepsy are more likely than others to suffer from depression. Many of the anti-epileptic medications, including one I took every day, carry Black Box Warnings alerting prescribers that patients may experience depressed mood or suicidal thoughts while taking the medication. Scientists have wondered for years whether the effects of abnormal electrical activity in the temporal and frontal lobes have long-term effects on mood, cognition, and ability to complete tasks of daily living. The fact is that living with the anticipation that seizures may appear at any moment sometimes brought me to my knees. No medication was needed to simulate that truth.

I learned to keep the dark thoughts and despair away by surrounding myself with as much beauty and grace as possible. I was blessed with beautiful children and a husband who loved and supported me through everything. The toothless grin of my younger son or the joyful skipping of my three-year-old were more potent than a bottle of Prozac to blast my blues away. A job that challenged and inspired me helped as well.

But as soon as I found a comfortable professional niche and our family was growing, I slipped into a slurry of frustration and discontent more often. There were fewer distractions to help me forget the seizures and the uncertainty that travelled with me like a leech to tender flesh. Previously, med school, residency, pregnancy, and caring for infants kept my mind occupied and hopelessness just outside my reach. Our children would get older, my patients would come and go, but epilepsy threatened to stay.

I learned to transform my children's radiant energy into my tonic. Their love created the elevator out of my abyss and the constant breath of fresh air in my uncertain life.

* * *

E

The word "epilepsy" is derived from the Greek verb *epilambanem*, which means "to take hold of or to seize." A common misconception is that patients either suffer recurrent grand mal seizures and live a life imprisoned by them, or patients are able to take a daily medication and have no seizures, no side effects, and no impact on their daily life.

The unfortunate truth is that in between the severely affected and the optimally controlled groups, there's a large cohort of patients exactly like me. Many of us have temporal lobe epilepsy, some have post-traumatic epilepsy from head injuries sustained in combat, and some have recurrent seizures of unknown etiology. Most of us are trying our best to live normal lives despite the constant threat of seizures and potent medications.

As the population of patients living with epilepsy has soared to 65 million people worldwide, an increasing amount of research has been done on the long-term outcome and health-related quality of life of patients with epilepsy. The research has focused on how the presence of seizures can affect other vital aspects of everyday life such as cognition, memory, mood, relationships, employment, fertility, and life expectancy.

Despite anti-epileptic drug treatment, up to one-third of patients diagnosed with any type of epilepsy continue to have seizures. Patients with drug-resistant temporal lobe epilepsy are at especially high risk for difficulty with memory and mood disorders such as depression and anxiety. This, in turn, leads to impairments in quality of life and increased risk for death.

Patients with evidence of scarring of the hippocampus on MRI are more likely than others without a defined lesion to have improvement in their seizures after surgical resection. However, other studies have shown that patients with documented structural brain abnormalities such as hippocampal scarring or atypical development of the cerebral cortex are more likely to develop medication resistant epilepsy.[26]

Multiple researchers have shown that recurrent seizures and associated side effects have a strong adverse effect on health-related quality of life. In fact, the effects of epilepsy are determined not only by the seizures themselves, but also by the meaning ascribed to the condition by a patient's social environment.[27] When patients with epilepsy encounter prejudiced attitudes, stereotypes, and erroneous beliefs from members of the community, the stigma associated with epilepsy may be more disabling than the seizures themselves. In many other cases, adverse medication effects may explain more variance in the quality of life than any other variable in patients with medication-resistant epilepsy.[28]

For patients who've had epilepsy surgery to remove a seizure focus, a long history of seizures prior to epilepsy surgery is associated with a higher risk of relapse. And even for those who achieve seizure control, cognitive dysfunction may not be reversible. Although many patients experience some post-operative seizures after a temporal lobectomy, the time to the first seizure from the time of surgery predicts long-term outcome. A shorter latency to the time of the first post-operative seizure is associated with poorer results.[29]

36
2008

WE FOUND OUT we were pregnant with our third child on a cool fall day in 2008. I shared the news with Andrew by presenting him with a furniture catalog dog-eared to the page depicting children's bunk beds. Our third pregnancy was carefully planned after prolonged conversations about benefits versus risks, discussions of ways to protect myself and a new baby, and whether adoption might be a safer choice for all of us. In the end, Andrew and I studied the perfect faces and brilliant minds of Alex and Will and decided to take our chances again.

News that I was expecting always came with conflicting emotions. I was excited for a new baby (we hoped for a girl), but afraid of the effects my medications may have on the baby's development. After two previous rocky pregnancies, I worried that my elevated hormones would provoke seizures, and wondered how another child would alter our family dynamics.

The first person I told about my pregnancy other than Andrew was my neurologist, Dr. Rodgers. I began the gradual process of increasing my medications to adjust for my increasing body weight several weeks later. At first I didn't notice anything new or different. Then slowly, as weeks turned to months and my abdomen swelled, my quick auras became more frequent despite the higher doses of medication.

Finally, one night, just like boiling water in a pressure cooker, the simmering electricity overflowed. I was jolted from sleep by the terrifying feeling that accompanied my complex partial seizures. My left hand clenched the bed sheets repetitively and my lips smacked an ominous rhythm. I was filled with a sense of foreboding when the small seizure receded. I turned to wake Andrew. A pointed elbow to the ribs finally roused him.

"Wha. . ." he mumbled then sat up in bed abruptly. "Are you OK?"

"I've just had a little seizure," I explained. "Can you stay up with me for a while to keep me company?" I hoped that if I avoided the wake-to-sleep transition, the time when I was more prone to seizures, my irritable brain would calm down.

"Of course." Andrew curled me in his arms. "Tell me what happened."

I described the typical small seizure and soon drowsiness covered me like a thick blanket. The clock by my bedside indicated that it was 2 A.M. "Good night," I murmured.

"I'm right here, Kristin," Andrew affirmed, pulling me closer. "Good night."

Then there were voices.

"Kristin?"

"Do you think she can hear me?"

"Kristin?"

A metallic sound followed, the click of a metal box opening. Someone grabbed my hand and pinched my lifeless finger. The dead weight of my arm returned to the bed, limp, as if it were disconnected from the rest of my body.

"Kristin? Can you open your eyes?"

I mustered a one-eyed glance at my surroundings. I was in my bed, but the lights were on. There was a uniformed stranger in the room calling my name. Oxygen tubing rested in my nose and a Band-Aid stuck on the spot on my finger where they'd checked my blood sugar.

"You've had a seizure," the kind voice said. "How are you feeling?"

Damn.

As usual, I could hear and partially understand the voices but my ability to respond lagged far behind. "Tired," I garbled with effort. I drifted back into the void again.

The voices around me paused briefly, then continued their narrative. One voice belonged to Andrew, the others were strangers. "We'll give her some time to wake up," a stranger stated. "Do you think she'll want to go to the hospital?"

Andrew responded, "No. We've been through this before. We know there's not much the hospital can do for her other than what you're doing now. Besides, Kristin is a doctor and she knows when to ask for help."

If only my M.D. could make me better.

A warm hand jostled mine. "Kristin? Can you open your eyes?"

I complied as best as I could.

"Do you want to go to the hospital?"

I gently shook my head. I just wanted to go to sleep.

Later, I heard the clang of the metal box closing, a *whoosh* of air as the oxygen prongs were removed from my nostrils, and the murmur of far-away voices on the EMS radio.

The next time I awoke, the room was dark. Andrew was back in his spot next to me, and the house was quiet. I adjusted my pillow and winced at the full-body ache that followed each grand mal seizure. Andrew pulled closer to me when I moved the covers.

"Are you alright?" he whispered.

"Yes, I will be."

I fell asleep and basked in the knowledge that no matter how tumultuous my life could be, I was safe with Andrew by my side.

*   *   *

After the first grand mal seizure of my third pregnancy, Dr. Rodgers recommended that I keep diazepam (trade name Valium) at home to stop any seizure activity in the future. I felt sheepish the next day when I went to pick up the medication. One of the benefits of working with a primary care medical group was that we provided excellent and convenient health care to many. One of the drawbacks of this was that my health insurance required that I seek health care in the same facilities where I worked. The same pharmacists who filled prescriptions written by Dr. Seaborg each day dispensed increasing amounts of medicine to patient Dr. Seaborg each month.

Yet the pharmacy staff was always very professional. They greeted me with a smile and took my bottles of medication off the shelf before I had the chance to announce my name. I cared for several of their children and grandchildren as patients. Stops for medication refills often turned into prolonged visits with updates about our extended primary care family.

Still, when the pharmacists handed over more and different anti-epilepsy medicines, I wondered what they were thinking. The staff never asked about my diagnosis or current course, but they must've discerned that I was struggling with uncontrolled seizures. Since they knew I ingested multiple mind-numbing medications, I worried that they questioned my competency as a physician.

Dr. Rodgers prescribed the liquid form of Valium because it works quickly and was the most likely to stop a seizure. Valium is a controlled medication that cannot be electronically prescribed, so I brought a written prescription to the pharmacy to have it filled.

The normally friendly pharmacist, Kate, looked at me with raised eyebrows when I handed her my prescription. The instructions called for me to "take 1 mL as needed up to 4 mL per day." There was no additional information to describe what "as needed" meant and there are many medical uses for Valium. My prescription could be for anxiety. It could be for withdrawal from alcohol or for muscle spasm. Or, I could need the Valium for seizures.

Kate studied the prescription and signature of the doctor who wrote it and I tried to melt into my coat and disappear. She looked up and caught my eyes with hers after what seemed like forever. Though she was trying, she had a hard time hiding her suspicion. "I have to look at your chart," she explained. "This isn't the typical way we use this medication."

"Yeah, sure, that's fine." I tried to appear nonchalant, although I was deeply ashamed. I wished there were a place where I could get my medicines that didn't send the doctor and patient parts of me on a collision course, or leave me feeling humbled and insecure.

I took a magazine from a nearby rack and held it as high and close to my face as I could while I waited for my prescription. I saw two of my patients enter the waiting area and turned my body closer to the wall. I didn't want to explain my reasons for lingering in the pharmacy waiting room so it was best not to be seen at all. Finally, I got my medicine and exited the building quickly and quietly like a raccoon caught foraging in the night.

I'd spent most of my life trying to fit in. Epilepsy "outed" me in a variety of unwelcome ways, like a violent storm roaming the clear blue sky. I was the guest at a party who asked for a soda instead of wine; the doctor in the prescription pick-up line trying to hide; the patient with the atypical prescriptions wishing for something generic; and the epileptic with recurrent seizures who desperately tried to pretend that they didn't exist.

I met Andrew in the car and we slowly pulled out of the pharmacy parking lot, averting my eyes from two colleagues who were walking back into the clinic after lunch. One colleague limped from cerebral palsy and I knew the other wore a breast prosthesis after a mastectomy several years ago. Perhaps fitting in was a myth of the invulnerable, underexposed, and insincere. We were all outcasts from our superficial world of perfection.

37

THE TWENTY-WEEK ULTRASOUND confirmed our hopes that
our third baby was a girl. I rejoiced in her clean bill of health and
immediately started buying everything pink. I was convinced that
our little girl couldn't sleep with old blue blankets in the crib. She
needed new pink ones. Her pacifier ring would be pink, as well as
the myriad barrettes I bought to put in her nonexistent hair.

Three months remained before my due date, and I felt great. The
boys were excited about the arrival of their new baby sister, and I
had a great time decorating the nursery and dreaming about raising
a little girl.

Then, like a low-lying mountain, epilepsy bumped up against my
happy world. This time, though, I was prepared.

The circumstances were almost identical to before. I woke from a
deep sleep as a complex partial seizure was building. I lay under the
protective down comforter after the seizure abated and listened to
the owls hoot greetings to one another outside. Unwilling to chance
another grand mal seizure, I woke Andrew.

"Can you help me get my medicine?" I asked. "I just had a seizure
and I'm not sure I'll dose it right on my own."

We rolled out of bed and met in the harsh, unnatural light of the
bathroom. I shielded my eyes while Andrew read from the bottle
of Valium.

"Take 4 milliliters of this," he instructed. He drew up the first milliliter.

The medication tasted like my grandfather's potent whiskey. It burned down my throat and offered comfort in knowing that I was doing everything I could to stop another seizure. We went back to bed, nestled in the warmth of our blankets and pillows and drifted back to sleep.

The Valium wasn't enough to quell my irritable neurons. The scene and seizure that followed, however, were less dramatic. There were no paramedics, no oxygen, and no cackling radios. Instead, I woke the next morning with a gash in my tongue, a gripping headache, and total body soreness. Andrew informed me in a mater-of-fact tone, "You had a grand mal seizure last night."

Everything after that made sense. I didn't remember the seizure, but its calling cards—the soreness, confusion, and tongue biting— were hard to ignore.

"I don't call the paramedics anymore," he explained. "I just watched the clock, held onto you, and prayed that the seizure would end."

And so it was in our marriage as it was with all things. We determined what tasks we could handle, managed challenges in whatever way we could, and prayed that God would help us through the rest.

* * *

One of my favorite things about being a pediatrician is caring for the small babies and meeting with first-time parents. In many ways, new parents are like children. Some are independent, some need their hands held through every new challenge, and all of them grow, change, and mature with the parenting experience.

Kari was a first-time mother of a beautiful boy named Charlie. At six months old, Charlie had a perfect round head with a shock of curly-Q Charlie Brown hair and large blue eyes resting in his face like porcelain saucers. I was Charlie's pediatrician from his first day of life and watched his scrawny newborn legs blossom into fat, doughy sausages, just as his cranky newborn fussiness emerged into smiling baby happiness. As a first-time mom, Kari had a consistent list of questions for me at each well-child visit. The questions ranged from as simple as "What should we expect next?" to "What educational toys should I buy to make Charlie smarter?"

I enjoyed visits with Kari and Charlie because Charlie was a gorgeous and happy boy and also, because it was fun to watch Kari grow in her confidence as a parent. But one afternoon the pair came to see me, and Kari was clearly alarmed.

"I don't know what's wrong with him!" Kari worried. "He hasn't been himself!"

I noted the deep lines etched in Kari's forehead. She bounced Charlie nervously on a quivering knee while he looked at me and smiled his tremendous grin, toothless and wide and brimmed with drool.

"Can you tell me more?" I asked.

Kari took a deep, shaky breath. "A couple of days ago I noticed that Charlie had a bit of a runny nose. His snot was clear and runny and Charlie was pretty happy otherwise, so I assumed he caught his first cold."

Charlie cooed in agreement as his mother talked.

"Then last night," she continued, "he cried every time I tried to put him down and he's been *very* fussy today. He's not interested in feeding this morning and he had a gigantic diaper of diarrhea just before we came here."

"Okay," I replied. "Is there anything else you've noticed?"

Kari grimaced and sniffed and looked away quickly as she fought back tears. "I'm just so worried about him!" she choked. I handed her a tissue. "Charlie's never acted like this before!"

Kari talked through her tears as I began an exam. "I went back to work two weeks ago and Charlie started day care. Since then, it's been one thing after another. First, he didn't want to take the bottle while I was away. Then, he didn't want to nap at daycare. Now, he's got this cold or virus or whatever it is and it's making me crazy!"

I felt Charlie's neck and looked in his mouth. Kari talked on.

"To top it off, my job is more demanding than it's ever been before. I feel like I'm doing a terrible job in the office and a terrible job of being a parent, too." Kari's tears flowed freely.

My exam completed, I rolled my chair away from Charlie so I could look directly at Kari. "Well, I've got good news for you, then," I said softly. "Charlie is okay. All of his symptoms can be attributed to these." I pointed to his lower gum line where two brand new teeth were erupting.

Kari slumped into her baby with relief and we had a good laugh together. Thankfully, it wasn't meningitis, an overwhelming infection, or any nightmare crisis that took shape in her mind.

Kari and Charlie taught me a lesson that I could easily apply to my own life. I spent a significant amount of time overanalyzing every fleeting unusual feeling, each headache that lasted too long, every floating wisp of lightheadedness, and worried that these were certain signs I was about to have a seizure. Kari, who'd recently returned to work rattled and overwhelmed, found it easy to permit her internal stress to alter her view of the world. Similarly, when I was more tired than usual or more frazzled by events at work or at home, I, too, was plagued by a soundtrack of fear that played in repetition on the outer edge of my consciousness.

I needed to step out of my pattern of worry. Worrying about everything couldn't change the course of events. Over-analysis only made life's irregularities more ominous and omnipotent than they probably were.

The door to the exam room opened and Kari exited with a happy baby bundled in a blue snowsuit. "Thank you," she said, touching my hand.

"Of course," I responded "Thank *you*."

Kari looked at me quizzically before she turned to head toward the exit. "See you next week!" she called over her shoulder, probably meaning it.

38
2009

KALLISTA ANN SEABORG was born on an early summer morning at 3:05 A.M. She was 6 pounds 13 oz., 19 inches long and had an adorable pointy nose that ran up to her round, voluminous eyes and a perfect, bare head that was, in the words of our obstetrician, "bald as a Lutheran minister."

Unlike the day Will was born, there were few reminders of epilepsy in the delivery room. Perhaps in an attempt not to lure the devil, the doctors avoided mentioning seizures or epilepsy by name. When I met the OB resident, he asked, "Tell me about your, um, you know…" My obstetrician kept an IV in a day longer than usual "in case you do anything funny…"

Regardless, when Kalli arrived, we were thrilled and relieved to meet our perfect little girl. After the remnants of childbirth were cleaned up and the hospital staff left the room, I nursed her in the pre-dawn quiet of a new day and admired her. I ran my fingers over her head, her back, her legs and arms and thanked God yet again for this flawless human being entrusted to us. I caressed her tiny rib cage and envisioned eventual gymnastics outfits, leotards, and ballet tutus spread over her graceful torso. I swallowed my worry for Will, who was no longer our youngest child, and for Alex, who suddenly had even more responsibility as the oldest of three.

We took Kalli home on a rainy day with clouds so thick they painted the horizon lavender and green. A strong wind blew the trees back and forth in greeting to our new addition. Soon after we arrived at the house, Kalli fussed and cried with hunger. Will walked up to his new sister with two fingers planted in his mouth and another excavating his nose. Innocently, he asked, "Can you please put her back in your tummy?"

I laughed and pulled Kalli close. She began to nurse and her crying stopped. Will crawled next to me and snuggled close. Alex crept up and nuzzled on my other side. We were going to be just fine.

* * *

It felt like I was starting over when I went back to visit Dr. Rodgers after Kalli was born. The zonisamide, keppra and occasional Valium didn't stop my seizures during pregnancy nor after I delivered the baby. Dr. Rodgers studied my chart along with the double-page sheet that listed all my medications, dosages, and length of each therapy. He looked at me over the top of the blue card-stock and considered what to try next.

"How about oxcarbamezepine? Have you tried that one?" he asked, squinting at the page.

"That was the medicine that gave me double vision. I don't think I want to try that again."

"O.K., how about lamotrigine?" I could only see his quizzical eyes over the mound of paper that detailed my medical history.

"I stopped that a few years ago because it wasn't working anymore."

"Not a good choice then." Dr. Rodgers grimaced and flipped back through the chart to the first few pages. "How about carbamazepine? It looks like you had some success with carbamazepine in the past."

"Yeah, I think I did." I remembered my early college years when my seizures were still infrequent. "Let's try that again."

I was starting over.

Dr. Rodgers stepped out of the room to summon the pharmacist to inform me how to transition between medications. After he left, I inspected the exam room I'd visited for the previous ten years. Though the location of the clinic was on a different floor of the hospital than before, the décor was almost identical to a decade previously. There were still pictures of a disembodied brain hanging on one wall, next to a color-coded anatomical map detailing the areas of varying structure and function. There was the familiar poster with large pictures of many anti-epileptic drugs. I could identify at least four distinct pills that'd graced my medicine cabinet at one time or another. And there were the two thinly upholstered chairs arranged next to the desk, one of which I sat in nervously.

Although I'd visited this clinic several times a year for a decade, I came with a renewed sense of hope every time. Prior to each visit, I dreamt that Dr. Rodgers would inform me of a new "fix" for seizures that would work for me. At the same time, I feared he might affirm that I would never find a cure. Hope was both extinguished and renewed inside the plain clinic walls. This time, I was starting a new medication that wasn't really new at all. Despite my best efforts to steer off the path of chronic illness, I'd come full circle.

Dr. Rodgers walked in the room with Mitch Caros and interrupted my reverie. Mr. Caros greeted me like we were old friends which, in a sense, we were. He gave me precise instructions as to how I would slowly increase the dose of my new medication and then eventually taper off the other two. I studied the sheet of paper where he was taking notes and focused on the several-week period where he suggested that I take three very strong anti-epileptic drugs at the same time. I wasn't sure how I would tolerate taking three medications at once. Mr. Caros offered me another piece of paper with his direct phone number in case I had questions or concerns during the transition. Even he wasn't sure if the switch would be tolerable.

On my way to the first floor exit, I stepped onto an elevator already filled with a team of pediatric residents and attending physicians, all of whom I knew from my time working at the hospital. I tried to look down and avert my eyes, but they knew who I was, and they knew I didn't work there anymore. I shoved my paperwork and prescriptions into my pocket and offered a forced smile.

"Hi Kristin!" one attending physician effused. "What brings you here?"

"Uh, hi Katie," I stumbled. "I was just in for a doctor's appointment."

"Oh, great." An awkward silence followed. Four floors had never moved so slowly. "Everything okay?"

"Oh, yeah. For sure."

The pack of residents, all draped in long white coats with pockets loaded with manuals and medical tools, studied their feet attentively. Finally, a soft *ping!* and the doors to the elevator opened. I pushed out into the cool hospital lobby. My face was burning.

I could've been in for an OB/GYN appointment, right? Didn't they have offices on the fourth floor? Or maybe they thought I was coming to see the cardiologist? No, their offices were in a different section of the hospital. In fact, the only adult clinic in the H section of the fourth floor was the Neurology and Epilepsy clinic. My interaction with Dr. Cohen years before made me think that epilepsy was an unacceptable unknown for physicians.

My heart sank. After years of careful professional disguise, my secret was again discovered. I processed my embarrassment and simultaneously felt frustrated that I had to hide anything at all. Epilepsy isn't a crime, but an illness. I'm not more or less of a person because I have seizures. I'm not a better or worse pediatrician because I take daily medications. I was tired of hiding behind a veil of carefully constructed normalcy.

I carried my new prescription to my friends at the pharmacy and waited behind a magazine while it was filled. I glowered as I drove home through the warm autumn evening, too tough to abandon old habits, too fragile to come out of the shadows. I studied Mr. Caros' carefully written instructions and vowed that one day I would break the chains of misconception and live fully and honestly as the broken person I was, imperfections and all.

39

THE MEDICATION SWITCH was almost as brutal as I feared. Each week, I slowly added a little more carbamazepine to my witch's brew of zonisamide and keppra. I slipped further into a sludge of exhaustion, dizziness, and nausea as the carbamazepine dose increased. My vision was blurry every time I adjusted my gaze and my brain felt as if it were floating in a directionless fog. It took genuine effort to keep my eyes open all day and even more effort to sound professional and intelligent at work. The kids hid their concerned expressions when Mommy went to bed at their bedtime every night, 8 P.M.

Although people surrounded me all day, I felt completely alone. Alex, Will, and Kalli depended on me as a source of strength in their lives so I feigned energy and enthusiasm even when I had none. I couldn't tell Andrew how I felt; he would beg me to stay home and stop working until I felt better. I didn't want to worry my parents, and I didn't want to concern my colleagues. On my darkest days of medication-induced stupor, I agonized that things may never get better.

Thankfully, the day finally came when I reached my target dose of carbamazepine and I began weaning off the other medicines. My eyes were the first things to improve. On high doses of three medications, I had trouble with blurry vision when I looked from a patient to the computer or if I looked quickly from a computer screen to the keyboard. Slow accommodation, the optometrist told me. A little less zonisamide and my ability to accommodate returned to normal. Next, my nausea let up. Then, the dizziness decreased. When I eventually weaned back to carbamazepine alone, the fatigue lessened, though never fully disappeared.

One Sunday evening in the midst of my medication switch, I read the Sunday paper after the kids went to bed. Even when they were asleep, the walls of my house reverberated with remnants of the chaos and clamor from the day. But when I sat in my basement office and watched the fire in the gas fireplace, a sliver of calm trickled in.

I turned the pages of the newspaper while hardly paying attention. As usual on Sunday night, my mind was occupied with the events of the coming week. Through my distraction and exhaustion, a headline caught my eye and made my heart race.

OBACK ADVISOR DAVID AXELROD TO SPEAK AT FUNDRAISER IN MADISON

Presidential advisor David Axelrod will speak in Madison on May 9 during a fundraiser for epilepsy research. Axelrod will be the keynote speaker at the event for Citizens United for Research in Epilepsy, or CURE, which Axelrod's wife founded. The Axelrods have a daughter with epilepsy.

This is the third year Madison Friends of CURE has held the fundraiser, according to organizer Eileen Sutula.

The event runs from 5:30-7:30 p.m. at Monona Terrace. For more information, see www.cureepilepsy.org.

— *Wisconsin State Journal* March 16, 2010

I stared at the paper for a long time. I envisioned the opportunity to meet and talk to others about epilepsy without feeling embarrassed. It was a chance to step out of my artificial shell and begin living outside of the shadows.

I swallowed my nerves and turned on my laptop to compose a simple email to the contact person listed on the website.

Dear Eileen,

My name is Kristin Seaborg. I am a pediatrician, a mother of three, and a patient with epilepsy. I am interested in attending the upcoming CURE event on May 9th. Could you please tell me how I could obtain tickets to this event?

Sincerely,
Kristin Seaborg, MD

I studied the email and revised it a multitude of times. Should I include the 'MD' or did that seem pretentious? Was it necessary that she know I'm a mother? Did I write in a kind-enough tone or did I sound demanding? I almost never spoke of epilepsy to anyone besides my doctors and immediate family. It was a big step to send a random email into cyberspace in hope that it would reach someone who would understand.

Before I could think about it anymore, I clicked Send and listened to the computer-generated *woosh* that indicated the message was beyond my retrieval. With a belly full of uneasiness and hope in my heart, I went upstairs to check on the kids.

It was the beginning of a new era.

I slept fitfully that night. I was both excited and petrified that Eileen, whoever she was, might get my email and want to talk more. The next morning, there was a message waiting for me.

Dear Kristin~

Thanks for your email. I would love to meet with you to tell you more about the upcoming event and Madison Friends

*of CURE. Could we meet for coffee sometime? I'm sure my
husband, Tom, would also be very interested in meeting you.*

Warmly,
Eileen

Excited by her response, I closed my email and did the most log-
ical thing I could think of: I Googled Tom and Eileen Sutula.

Eileen Sutula was founder and leader of the Madison chapter
of Citizens United for Research in Epilepsy (CURE), an international nonprofit organization that raises funds to support epilepsy
research. She ran the growing Madison organization and raised
tens of thousands of dollars to fund neuroscientists throughout the
country in their efforts to learn more about the pathophysiology and
treatment of seizures. Tom Sutula was the chair of the University of
Wisconsin Department of Neurology and a neurologist who specialized in epilepsy. They were a friendly and successful couple with
significant local influence.

We arranged to meet at a local coffee shop. In the two weeks
between the exchange of emails and our date for coffee, I imagined
what it would be like to talk openly about epilepsy outside of my
home or Dr. Rodgers' office for the first time.

The day of my first meeting with Eileen and Tom, I woke with
the emerging light. My children wandered out of their rooms in
their usual fashion, one by one, with hair tousled and eyes squinting
to adjust to the morning brightness.

Will and Alex, adorned in their truck and train footie pajamas, lay
on the floor of our bedroom while I showered. "What are you doing
today, Mommy?" Alex asked.

"Oh, not much," I fibbed. I came out from behind the steam-
coated wall of the shower and toweled off. "I'm going to meet with
my friends for coffee and then I have to go to work."

"Who are your friends?" Will piped up, his mouth full of graham
crackers and apple juice.

I didn't really know how to answer.

"Just some friends who are involved in something I'm interested in," I said, as non-specifically as possible, hoping they'd move on.

Alex, the perpetually inquisitive and curious member of our family, persisted. "What are you interested in, mommy?"

"Nothing important, sweetie. Now, it's time to get ready for school." A chorus of grumbling rose from the boys' throats as they reluctantly collected their sippy cups of juice and tiny bowls of crackers and headed back to their room.

I dressed quickly, and soon was seated next to Andrew in our black S.U.V., headed to the suburban coffee shop where we planned to meet. In early April, which can be considered the very beginning of spring or the very end of winter in Wisconsin, the days grow longer but the sun still rises over a cold landscape each morning. That morning, a crystalline layer of frost covered the greening blades of grass, reflecting a thousand tiny rainbows in the prisms of frozen dew. We drove through prisms of sparkling light and ephemeral wisps of fog.

The scene transformed into something slightly less majestic when we pulled into the strip-mall parking lot. Andrew dropped me off next to a stubborn, browning clump of snow in the sparsely populated lot. I checked my watch. Happy to be early, I had time to get coffee on my own and calm the quivering inside.

My hand shook when I accepted the steaming cup of Joe from the barista at the counter. My involuntary, visceral reaction to the upcoming meeting surprised me. Though cognizant of my efforts to hide my vulnerability, I never fully appreciated how all-encompassing I believed my performance needed to be. As much as I privately thought about seizures, side effects, and my prognosis, I unwittingly spent as much mental energy hiding my thoughts, my fears, and my Achilles heel. I didn't understand how liberating honesty would be.

After a short time, an unfamiliar woman scurried through the door, and scanned the small cafe as if she were looking for someone. Her thick winter coat doubled the size of her petite frame and her expression, even from a distance, was compassionate and kind. I started to rise to beckon her to my table, but she was already headed my way with a broad smile.

"Eileen?" I extended my hand to shake hers.

"Kristin. It's such a pleasure to meet you." She studied me with perceptive eyes as we headed to the small table at the back of the shop. "Tom had an early meeting, but he'll be on his way as soon as he can."

Eileen put her coat on the back of a chair and excused herself to get some coffee. I sat quietly in my seat and sipped my drink. I steadied my shaking hands around the warm mug. Within moments, Eileen was back. Rising tentacles of steam emanated from her drink and surrounded her face in a ghostly manner. She took a seat across from me and didn't waste time.

"Tell me your story."

For the next hour, I told Eileen, and then Tom, about my journey with epilepsy. While I talked, a sense of emancipation grew as they listened without judgment. Tom, although a well-known researcher and prominent leader in neuroscience, talked in a gentle tone and asked probing questions about what it was like to practice medicine and live with epilepsy. He listened as if my story mattered to him. Unlike most of my friends and family, neither one of them used euphemisms for "seizures" or avoided saying the word "epilepsy." It was a relief to finally acknowledge what I'd sequestered for so long without worrying that I would be viewed differently in the end.

We met and talked for almost two hours. Tom and Eileen told me more about CURE and the epilepsy community in Madison. After we exchanged contact information and said goodbye, I walked outside with a smile on my face and a confidence I hadn't known. I relished in a new sense of hope and promise. Stone by stone, the wall was crumbling.

40
2010

I WOKE IN THE MORNING several months later with a feeling of expectation. Coffee in one hand and shaving with the other, Andrew asked, "Are you nervous about your appointment today?"

"No more than usual," I responded, knowing that the news I was bringing to the doctor was far from the seizure-free existence we were striving for.

My mind drifted through the previous months while I dried my hair. I remembered our tenth anniversary and a walk down Michigan Avenue in Chicago, my heart filled with love and contentment, suddenly interrupted by the old, unwelcome waves of heat, swallowing, and confusion. There was the day in clinic in the fall when I had a seizure in an exam room. I was listening to a newborn's heart when my left hand involuntarily clenched the stethoscope before compulsory lip smacking and recurrent swallowing were all I knew. And there was the evening when I was standing in the kids' bathroom, combing Alex's hair before bed. My left hand clamped his head like a vice until he complained. I was too immersed, confused, and overpowered by the seizure to remove it. Andrew gently took my hand and beckoned me to the floor until the seizure pulled away like waves at the shore. The list went on and on. About every two weeks, epilepsy reared its ugly head and the monster within me woke.

Visits to U.W. Hospital always left me with conflicting emotions. The large, awkward building housed both my former employer and my persistent health care providers. So much had changed, and still so little. I ran into several former colleagues on the walk to the neurology department. I had to wonder if, when I was dressed in casual clothes, they were more apt to see through my outer physician persona and notice the insecure patient inside.

Dr. Rodgers surprised me with his thoughts after I reviewed my seizure history from the previous six months. Though I'd learned to cope with it, he thought that one to two seizures every two weeks was unacceptable. I suppose in some corner of my overactive mind I'd settled for a life pocked by intermittent seizures. Dr. Rodgers spoke first about increasing my current medication but then, unbelievably, maybe eventually considering another brain surgery.

He studied my post-operative MRI and thought out loud. "Well, you already have that visual field defect," he said. "There probably is a little active tissue here... maybe another seizure focus... and I suppose we can remove that without harming you." He pointed to area on the MRI adjacent to the gaping hole that used to house my right temporal lobe. "You're probably not using those areas of your brain anyway."

Visions of weeks of pain, tests, hospital stays, and headaches loomed large. I wanted to scream: *I can't go through that again! My family depends on me! They can't see me sick and weak when I am supposed to be strong!*

With effort, I calmed my thoughts and attended to Dr. Rodgers again. He decided that the most appropriate first step would be to increase my dose of carbamazepine and follow-up in clinic in three months. We would continually re-assess the need for further procedures based on the status of my seizures.

After my appointment, I walked across the street to my favorite place on campus where, as an undergrad, I went when I sought peace and solitude. I ambled through the Picnic Point parking lot and walked onto the quiet path down the peninsula, losing myself in the vibrant vegetation. My feet pounded the dirt in time to the mantra in my mind: *I can't be sick. I have to be strong. My family depends on me.*

Doubt swam into the rhythm of my resolve. Did I not take my seizures seriously enough? I knew that emotional stress and sleep deprivation increased my risk of seizures yet I still led a stressful, exhausting life. Was it time to make a meaningful change? I'd read portions of the emerging body of medical literature hypothesizing that seizures beget seizures and recurrent seizures in adulthood could lead to eventual memory changes and loss. What kind of mother would I be if I couldn't remember the children's soccer games or dance classes or even the stories that shaped their childhood?

The cicadas pulsed a gentle beat while I walked through the tunnel of green trees. I stopped to admire the lake and the glistening Capitol dome not far beyond. A gull dove to capture a surface-swimming fish and a large, white swan navigated the waves as he swam through a path in the lily pads. I reflected on the beautiful, yet constantly changing and unpredictable path of nature and the previously elusive truth was finally clear.

I didn't know what to expect. Whether more medication and sedation would become necessary, additional surgery, or gradual intellectual decline, I couldn't plan the rest of my life as I had before. I must be like the gull and grasp opportunities as they appear. I needed to learn from the swan and swim through unexpected obstacles with grace. I had to enjoy every day and live in the moment because I'll never know what tomorrow will bring.

In the twenty years since I was diagnosed with epilepsy, my disease took many shapes. In turn, I've carried many labels. Complex partial. Surgically correctable. Recurrent. Intractable.

I wasn't curable, but I was still teachable. I stepped down from my vantage point over Madison and rested in the knowledge that I was still walking on this infinite journey. During my walk back along the peninsula, I gulped the green, humid air and allowed nature to teach me.

The rhythm of the lapping waves against the nearby shore demonstrated that even if I employed my most sophisticated methods of avoidance and denial, time marched on. The patches of rotting mossy grass and decomposing tree trunks in the small patches of forest nearby were a physical reminder that with each failure, there's opportunity for renewal. The delicate sounds of squirrels skittering up and down trees for nuts showed me that with perseverance, even the smallest and most vulnerable of us can succeed. When I stopped to watch a large beetle fan its wings on a nearby tree, I noticed the intricate red markings across its back and the iridescent elegance of its slowly undulating wings. The beetle revealed that if I looked closely, I can find beauty in even the ugliest of things.

Perhaps there's beauty in the way epilepsy taught me grace, gratitude, perseverance, strength, and hope. Maybe I needed to take this journey to become mindful of the blessings surrounding me. Perhaps only when forced to live with vulnerability and uncertainty could I learn to treasure and give thanks for the simplest of things. Maybe I learned to care for all aspects of each patient only after I was a patient myself. I resolved to live a purposeful life shaped by these truths.

I was at peace with epilepsy, peace moving in like the quiet after a storm. The fingers of acceptance and understanding tickled my strong will and it was no longer necessary to live in a shadow. Dual lives are for those who're ashamed. Concealed vulnerabilities are for those who're unwilling to accept that they're always vulnerable. It was time for me to lift the curtain and claim the irreparably damaged parts of me.

I was no longer ashamed.

41
2010

THE LARGE AUDITORIUM was about a third full, the green-cushioned chairs filled with a spattering of familiar faces and strangers. Papers rustled, a scattered cough answered by a lone sniffle. Several well-dressed adults walked the narrow aisles to search for an open seat in back. The air was filled with a soft buzz of expectation and curiosity.

I sat at the front table at the fourth annual Madison Friends of CURE event. I was one of a panel of speakers asked to speak about my experience or expertise in epilepsy. Last year, I'd attended as a wide-eyed visitor. Now, I was part of the tapestry. I'd come a long way in a year, but still not far enough. The seizures persisted, there was at least one more medication trial, and I remained reluctant to talk about epilepsy. It was time to make a change.

In the audience, Andrew stared up at me, sending strength and his courage. He knew more about my epilepsy than most, yet still, even from my husband, I hid many of my seizures and symptoms. My parents and Andrew's sat near the back and studied their programs. They all were familiar with my seizures but had no idea how they'd plagued me in recent years. There were two pediatric neurologists with whom I was professionally acquainted, but who had no idea that I had epilepsy. There were several friends we invited as guests; the Sutulas were there, of course, other new friends whom I'd came to know through CURE; and a handful of people I'd never seen before. After a lifetime, I was "coming out" for good.

I'd practiced my speech about one hundred times while driving to work or walking in the neighborhood. I was nervous about sharing my story, but when my turn came to step up to the podium, an unexpected calm washed over me.

This was where I belonged.

Slowly, but most definitely, sorrow and isolation lifted away as I spoke. My words brought catharsis to my injured soul and healed the loneliness and despair lingering around my disease. Once I shared my story, it was no longer mine to conceal and protect. I concluded my speech with a poem I wrote to explain what it's like to live with epilepsy.

> Living with epilepsy means that I know the distinctive scent of EEG glue as well as I know the scent of my children.
>
> Living with epilepsy means that I've learned how to fall asleep in MRI machines, wait patiently in doctors' offices, and perform neurological tests without prompting.
>
> Living with epilepsy means that I must not be the "Epileptic Patient" but rather "the patient with epilepsy." I cannot let the seizures own me.
>
> Living with epilepsy means that even some of my most significant days have been accompanied by seizures: the day I delivered my son, my tenth anniversary, Christmas Day, Thanksgiving.
>
> Living with epilepsy means that when the familiar sensations of a partial seizure appear, I find myself searching for a place to sit away from view in case the simple seizure leads to something more.
>
> Living with epilepsy means hiding my illness under a well-designed shroud, afraid that if others know that I have seizures they will lose their faith and trust in me.

Living with epilepsy means I examine my tongue each morning in the mirror to look for the characteristic bite that's my sign of a nocturnal seizure.

Living with epilepsy means learning to ignore the staggering fatigue that comes with each new medication trial and medication adjustment.

Living with epilepsy means that I can list almost every anti-seizure medication and its associated side effect profile. I have tried them all.

Living with epilepsy means that I treasure the mundane and hold these things as close as possible, for fear of losing them: driver's license, health insurance, life insurance.

Living with epilepsy means that I will consent to tests that turn off part of my brain, remain tethered to a wall with an extension cord for up to a week, and consent for removal of my entire temporal lobe in hopes for a cure that still eludes me.

Living with epilepsy means that I have created a handful of euphemisms to describe a seizure: head problem, not right, episode, incident.

Living with epilepsy means I feel compelled to join others like me and look down the long, dark road that I pray may ultimately lead to a cure.

I looked up to find Andrew's tear-stained face and met his eyes. I knew that together, we would watch our children with extreme care, worrying through their fevers and illnesses and praying that epilepsy wouldn't find them too. I knew that it was time to share my history with the children as well. My story had, after all, become part of the family tapestry that colors our past and hopes for the future.

The audience applauded when I finished reading. I took my seat, relieved. The monster, by revealing himself, could no longer own me.

2015

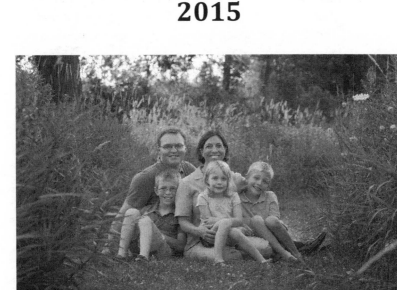

NOT FAR FROM MY HOUSE, there's a farmette that abuts a bucolic country road. When I'm lucky enough to steal a few moments away from the house in the evenings, I love to go for a walk and always make a point to pass the small farm. There's a weathered old barn next to a tidy house and small valley of luminescent green grass that grows right up to the gravel shoulder of the road.

Most evenings, two chocolate horses grace the valley and graze lazily in the field. Sometimes the horses hide behind the neighboring oak trees or stand in the shadows adjacent to the road. They huff as cars streak by and watch me with a curious eye if I speak to them. They stand tall and quietly resilient through the commotion of traffic, bikers, and trespassers.

I've come to think that the horses have a lot in common with my epilepsy. They are unwaveringly powerful, strong, and command respect. If untamed, they can overwhelm one quickly and threaten great danger. But when they're calm and hidden in the shadows, they're surprisingly magnificent and beautiful. Though epilepsy still taunts me, it's taught me to appreciate the beauty of my life and the value and strength of the human soul.

I still have seizures about once a month. They're the small, focal seizures that cause tingling in my left hand, repetitive swallowing, and lip movements. Now almost all of my seizures come in the middle of the night. They wake me from my slumber before I plunge again into an abyss of pulsing, tingling, and swallowing. The day before or after a seizure, I have many auras, but only I can tell.

My last grand mal seizure was six years ago, when I was pregnant with my daughter. The discussion that Dr. Rodgers and I had about another epilepsy surgery has been put to rest on the assumption that more resection may lead to serious detriments. At least for now, we've stopped the relentless switch from one anti-epilepsy medication to the next since changes are fraught with frustrating side effects but offer me little hope for a cure.

Our children are now eleven, nine, and six. They are fantastic miracles of energy who enlighten every day. Alex has become a gifted musician and can do math problems on par with my computer. Will loves to laugh and make others laugh and is perpetually stealing household items like scraps of wood, tape, and staples to make new creations. Kalli makes the word "ebullient" sound feeble as she jumps, sings and talks incessantly through her day. Quite often, I stare at all three of them and marvel that they are the products of nine months of intrauterine medications, chemicals, and seizures. All three kids have been taught how to call 9-1-1 and respond if Mommy has a seizure. So far my epilepsy hasn't cursed any of them. I hope it never will.

Andrew remains devoted and supportive despite all we've been through. He's become my champion and my unofficial agent, my cheerleader and confidant. He's read this book almost as many times as I and he's only edited a few lines from the role he plays. One of my goals in writing this memoir was to chronicle the love story that has blessed our marriage.

I try not to worry about when the next seizure is coming. I struggle not to spend time dwelling on my worst fear, that seizures are eroding my cognition and memory faster than they should. I catch myself watching our kids and wondering if they will remember how much I love them, how high I've hoped for them, and how hard I've tried to keep my illness from them.

Even after the worst of days, their smiling faces are proof that there is goodness in the world.

"Natural forces within us are the true healers of disease"
   ~ Hippocrates

References

[1] Goddard, G.V., McIntyre D. C., and Leech, C.K. (1969) A permanent change in brain function resulting from daily electrical stimulation. *Experimental Neurology,* 25, 295-300.

[2] Cavazos, J., Das, I., and Sutula, T. (1994) Neuronal loss induced in limbic pathways by kindling: Evidence for induction of hippocampal sclerosis by repeated brief seizures. *The Journal of Neuroscience,* 14(5), 3106-3121.

[3] Hermann, B., Seidenberg, M. (2007) Epilepsy and cognition. *Epilepsy Currents,* 7(1): 1-6.

[4] Kale, R. (1997) Bringing Epilepsy Out of the Shadows. *British Medical Journal* 315: 2-3.

[5] International League Against Epilepsy (2003) The History and Stigma of Epilepsy. *Epilepsia,* 44 (Suppl. 6): 12—14.

[6] From the German Epilepsy museum Kork—Museum for epilepsy and the history of epilepsy. http://www.epilepsiemuseum.de/alt/body_therapieen.html

[7] Moog FP, Karenberg, A. (2003) Between horror and hope: gladiator's blood as a cure for epileptics in ancient medicine. *Journal of History of Neuroscience*, 12(2): 137-43.

[8] Fidel, W., Leblanc, R., Nogueira de Alemeida, A. (2009) Epilepsy surgery: Historical highlights 1909-2009 *Epilepsia* 50 (Suppl. 3): 131-151.

[9] Weiser, HG. (1991) Selective amygdalohippocampectomy: indications and follow-up. *Canadian Journal of Neurologic Science* 18: 617—627.

[10] Magiorkinis, E., Sidiropoulou, K., and Diamantis, A. *Hallmarks in the History of Epilepsy: From Antiquity Till the Twentieth Century.* Office for the Study of History of Hellenic Naval Medicine, Naval Hospital of Athens, Greece.

[11] Pearce, JMS. (2002) Bromide, the first effective anti-epileptic agent. *Journal of Neurology and Neurosurgical Psychiatry*, 72: 412.

[12] Shorvon, S. (2009) Drug treatment of epilepsy in the century of the ILAE: The first 50 years, 1909-1958 *Epilepsia* 50 (Suppl. 3): 69-92.

[13] Nelson KB, Ellenberg JH. (1978) Prognosis in children with febrile seizures. *Pediatrics* 61 (5): 720-727.

[14] American Academy of Pediatrics Subcommittee on Febrile Seizures. (2008) Febrile Seizures: Clinical Practice Guideline for the long-term management of the child with simple febrile seizures. *Pediatrics* 121 (6): 1281-1286

[15] Sadleir JH, Scheffer, I. (2007) Febrile seizures. *British Medical Journal*, 334 (7588): 307-311.

[16]http://www.epilepsy.com/connect/forums/living-epilepsy-adults/epilepsy-stats-and-facts

[17] http://www.cureepilepsy.org/aboutepilepsy/facts.asp

[18] New Prayer Song Song, Pastor Gretchen Weller and The Pull: *Hadda Get Down to Get Up* (2002).

[19] Hoge C., McGurk D., Thomas J., Cox, A., Engel, C., Castro C. (2008) Mild Traumatic Brain Injury in U.S. Soldiers Returning From Iraq. *The New England Journal of Medicine*, 358; 5: 453-463.

[20] Pugh, MJ *et al.* (2015) The Prevalence of Epilepsy and Association with Traumatic Brain Injury in Veterans of the Iraq and Afghanistan Wars. *Journal of Head Trauma Rehabilitation* 30: 29-37.

[21] Schwab, K., Grafman, J., Salazar, A., Kraft, J. (1993) Residual Impairments and Work Status 15 Years After Penetrating Head Injury. *Neurology* 43 (1).

[22] Shukla, G., Prasad, A. (2012) The Natural History of Temporal Lobe Epilepsy: Antecedents and Progression. *Epilepsy Research and Treatment* Volume 2012.

[23] McIntosh, AM, Kalnins RM, Mitchell LA, Fabinyi GC, Briellmann RS, Berkovic SF (2004) Temporal Lobectomy: Long-term Seizure Outcome, Late Recurrence, and Risks for Seizure Recurrence *Brain* 127(Pt 9):2018-2030.

[24] Yerby, M., Lannon, S., Mittendorf, R. (1991) An Information Pamphlet for Women with Epilepsy. *Epilepsia* 32 (Suppl 6): S51-9.

[25] Sperling, M. (2001) Sudden unexplained death in epilepsy. *Epilepsy Currents* Vol 1, No. 1: 21-23.

[26] Kwan, P., Brodie, M. (2002) Refractory Epilepsy: A Progressive, Intractable, but Preventable Condition? *Seizure* 11: 77—84.

[27] Theo, P., Suurmeijer, M., Reuvekamp, M., Aldenkamp, B. (2001) Social functioning, psychological functionings, and quality of life in epilepsy. *Epilepsia*, 42 (9): 1160-1168.

[28] Perucca P., Gilliam F.G., Schmitz, B. (2009) Epilepsy Treatment as a Predeterminant of Psychosocial Ill Health. *Epilepsy Behavior*, 15 Suppl. 1: S46-50.

[29] Buckingham, S.E., Chervoneva, I., et al. (2010) Latency to first seizure after temporal lobectomy predicts long-term outcome. *Epilepsia*, 51 (10): 1987-93.

Photo Credits

Epilepsy Resources

I'm thrilled to announce that 100% of author royalties raised from this book will be donated to the **Citizens United for Research in Epilepsy**, or **CURE**. CURE is the largest private nonprofit worldwide that raises and donates money for research in epilepsy. You can learn more about CURE and make your own donation by visiting their website, www.cureepilepsy.org.

In addition to CURE, there are a multitude of nonprofit organizations dedicated to support those with epilepsy, educate others about epilepsy, and fund research in epilepsy. If you would like to learn more about epilepsy or support those who struggle with this frustrating disease, I recommend visiting any or all of the websites below.

Epilepsy Foundation of America
Works to ensure that people with seizures are able to participate in all of life's experiences and supports research for additional treatments and cure. www.epilepsy.com

American Epilepsy Society
A group of the world's leading epilepsy professionals who are experts in the most recent clinical research, technology, and treatments for epilepsy. www.aesnet.org

International League Against Epilepsy
"The world's preeminent association of physicians and other health professionals working towards a world where no person's life is limited by epilepsy." www.ilae.org

Danny Did Foundation
Advances awareness for Sudden Unexpected Death in Epilepsy (SUDEP) and promotes mainstreaming of seizure detection devices that may assist in preventing deaths caused by seizures. www.dannydid.org

Acknowledgments

When we moved from the condo to our house in the suburbs, I cleaned out my desk for the first time in years. Amidst piles of papers, notes from medical school, and keepsakes, I found four notebooks with four different attempts at telling my story. Though I didn't realize it at the time, this memoir has been percolating inside for years and waiting to be told.

I couldn't have come from a conglomeration of notes in scattered notebooks to publication without the support of my fantastic family, friends, health care providers, and colleagues. Specifically, I'd like to thank my parents, Ralph and Jo Gould, who gave me every opportunity available and opened dozens of doors of possibility during my formative years. My brothers, Jon and Paul Gould, taught me resilience through brotherly teasing and the importance of loyalty when times were tough.

Thank you to Andrew, of course, for loving me for who I am and for constructing a scaffolding of support that has held me upright through the most ominous of storms.

Thank you to my many skilled physicians, health care providers, and extended medical family who mastered the art of caring for my illness while simultaneously protecting my pride as a physician. To the many resident colleagues and life-long friends who were mentioned in this book, for the extra call you took, shoulders that I cried on, and times you were so much more than a colleague or a friend, I thank you.

For the handful of early readers: Tom and Eileen Sutula, Amanda Bryant, Jennifer Philbin, William Clark, and Andrew, thanks for your gentle guidance, thoughtful suggestions, and encouragement to muster through.

Thank you to Susan and David Axelrod for support of my story and for founding and breathing life into an organization that gives me hope and reason to believe that someday there will be more options for treatment of seizures.

Thank you to Justin Bogdanovitch and Susan Leon for their editorial expertise and for continuing to encourage me to write the best manuscript possible.

And, of course, thank you to Alexander, William, and Kallista Seaborg. For their patience with the days and nights that I stared at the computer instead of into their eyes and for giving me a thousand reasons to write and even more reasons to move on.

About the Author

Kristin Seaborg lives in Madison, Wisconsin with her husband, three adorable kids, and two overfed guinea pigs. She received her undergraduate degree from the University of Wisconsin and her M.D. from the University of Wisconsin School of Medicine and Public Health.

When not tending to her busy pediatrics practice or driving the kids to activities, Kristin finds time to write, garden, and drink a lot of coffee.

Website/Blog:
www.kristinseaborg.com

Twitter:
@kristinseaborg

Facebook:
Facebook.com/KristinSeaborgBooks

Snail Mail address:
7659 Summerfield Drive
Verona, WI 53593

Email:
kristinseaborg@gmail.com

MORE GREAT READS
FROM GRAVITY

Stigma Fighters Anthology by **Sarah Fader** (Anthology—Mental Health) Stigma Fighters is a non-profit mental health organization in Brooklyn, New York that seeks to give people living with mental illness a voice. This compilation of personal perspectives features essays from real people living with mental illness from around the globe.

Tea and Madness by **C. Streetlights** (Memoirs and Poetry) C. Streetlight's memoir, Tea and Madness, is a collection of prose and poetry separated into the seasons of her life. As her seasons change, she continues trying to find the balance of existing between normalcy and madness.

Fortitude: A PTSD Memoir by **Apryl Pooley** (Memoir) Fortitude describes Apryl's unrelenting attempts to hide her shame by escaping her mind and body, only to find that what she needed was to openly share her story and travel deep within herself to find the healing answers that were there all along.

Made in the USA
San Bernardino, CA
28 December 2015